Dynamic* Dentistry

Practice Management Tools and Strategy for Breakthrough Success

Linda Miles CSP, CMC

LiNK Publishing
Virginia Beach, VA

This and other practice management/staff development products are available by visiting the Linda Miles and Associates web site at www.dentalmanagementU.com or by calling toll free 800-922-0866.

Published by
Link Publishing
2788 Nestlebrook Trail
Virginia Beach, VA 23456

Publisher's Cataloging-in-Publication Data
Miles, Linda

Dynamic dentistry : practice management tools and strategy for breakthrough success / Linda Miles. --Virginia Beach, VA : Link, 2003

p ; cm.

ISBN 0-9658409-1-3

1. Dentistry—Practice—United States. 2. Dental offices—United States—Management. I. Title

RK58.5 .M55 2003 2002112209
617.6/0068—dc21 0301

Project coordination by Jenkins Group, Inc. * www.bookpublishing.com
Cover design by Ann Pellegrino
Cover photo by Eric Hinson of the office of Dr. Christopher E. Cooley
Interior design by Royce Deans

Printed in the United States of America

07 06 05 04 03 * 5 4 3 2 1

DEDICATION

This book is for dental teams everywhere, teams that have done so much to advance the dental profession since I was a young dental assistant years ago. The advancement of the concept of teamwork between dentists and their staff has enabled us to make offices more efficient and profitable and, most important, to greatly improve the quality of care we offer patients.

Teams of course are made up of individuals, and I want to acknowledge both. Specifically, I'd like to thank the dentists who have dedicated themselves to improving our profession through their commitment to ongoing professional education. Without them, there would be no dental profession. The strides they have made, in both their ability to operate a professional practice and the level of care they provide, continue to inspire me.

Most of all, this is a book for dental assistants, both business and clinical, and to hygienists in every practice in every corner of the country, for it is dental staff who have a special place in my heart. I gratefully acknowledge dental team members as the professionals who have played a huge role in helping shape the content of my seminars and all three of my books. I have watched and I hope in some small way advanced the evolution of the dental staff to an indispensable component of a successful dental practice.

Dynamic Dentistry is first and foremost for you.

CONTENTS

PREFACE

It takes patients about ten years to truly believe a dentist's clinical skills are exceptional. It takes them ten minutes to decide whether they want to be your patient and whether they will refer their family, friends, and colleagues to your practice.

If you're a dentist, this means that as important as your clinical skills are to building your practice, the quality of the experience your patients have before and after receiving care is equally important. It means you must put comprehensive, patient-friendly, and business savvy policies, procedures—and people!—in place and set a positive, welcoming tone for your entire office. And it means that your leadership and your personal example are critical, for statistics prove that employees treat patients the way their employer treats them.

If you're a member of a dental practice support team, the "ten-minute rule" exemplifies the pivotal role you play in building the practice. Your actions and attitude have a profound effect on those around you...for better or worse. You have the power to contribute to the growth and success of the practice and, by extension, to the growth and success of each team member. Clearly, you, along with every other member of the practice, have a personal stake in putting a lasting smile on each patient's face.

Easier said than done, as you know. The quality of the patient's experience depends upon many factors working in combination: the care they receive, the experience they have on the phone with you, the depth and clarity of the answers they get, the amount of time they spend in the reception area, and the way they are treated in an emergency to name just a few.

The Success Triangle

To put a genuine and lasting smile on each patient's face, a dental office must implement a powerful practice model I call the Success Triangle. On the first side of the triangle are the dentist's clinical skills. Nothing can replace those. On the second side are superior business skills that enable a practice to hum along each day at a productive clip. These include scheduling, collections, insurance, and recare for example.

At the base of the Success Triangle are communication skills. I put communication there because it is equal in importance to the other two and because it is also the foundation that supports them. Success does not happen without quality communication that assists and encourages every patient and every team member.

In short, successful communication is at the heart of every successful practice.

Dynamic Dentistry

When I began my position as an office administrator in 1976, fifteen years after my first dental assisting position, I quickly noticed how the total office environment—not just the quality of care patients received—factored into the practice's success. I started writing down the structure, policies, and procedures that worked best for us and eventually developed a practice management system for the office.

In 1984, while attending the Pankey Institute as a guest, I realized the entire dental team had to participate in a new way of thinking in order for the quality of care to change. Afterward, in 1985, I decided to devote myself to sharing my practice-building success strategies with as many dental professionals as possible. That was the inception of the LLM&A Dental Business Conference.

I've conducted hundreds of such workshops since. In the process, I've learned as much from the participants as they've learned from me. It's been a fabulous experience and a never-ending give and take of ideas, inspirations, and often hilarious anecdotes, not to mention the lifelong friends the many participants have become.

Dynamic Dentistry is the product of these many years of teaching, talking, laughing, and learning, and it is my great pleasure to share it with you. This book, my third on the topic of dental practice building, is for anyone who wants their practice to succeed and grow by delivering excellence in the total patient experience...to every patient, every day. I believe any dentist or dental employee who picks up this book will learn a minimum of fifteen new ways to significantly improve their practice.

Idea Sharing

Dentists and staff members derive the greatest benefit from my workshops when they attend together, and I readily encourage them to do so. For the same reasons, I recommend that everyone in your office read *Dynamic Dentistry*. Ideas are more easily accepted and implemented when everyone understands their origins. In addition, different people pick up on different ideas and strategies and offer their own perspectives, all of which makes for a more effective practice aimed at delivering a total patient experience that's upbeat and positive, and building patient relationships that last.

Of course I don't expect everyone in the office to buy a copy of *Dynamic Dentistry* (although I wouldn't object!), but I'd love to visit your practice one day and see my book on someone's desk, dog-eared, scribbled on, and not-so-gently used. I'll know then it was read, shared, collaborated, and even argued over. Nothing would make me happier.

The Fun Factor

In the last twenty years, the principles and techniques you're about to read have helped build many dental practices, some of which were on the brink of collapse because of poor finances, staffing problems, or patient attrition...tough business challenges you might expect a practice to face at one point or another.

But I've also seen many practices suffering from a vexing ailment called burnout. So many people arrive at one of my workshops looking tired and resigned and saying things like, "I think I've burned out" or "I'm just not having any fun." They're dreading every day, and may even be thinking about leaving the profession altogether.

I am a passionate crusader for putting the fun back in dentistry for everyone. In my seminars and in my consulting services, I help people remember this is a great profession. We help children, adults, seniors, and whole families feel better and smile more broadly. I tell them never to forget this, no matter what the day serves up. I get tremendous satisfaction seeing people leave my seminars with a smile on their face and a skip in their step. They've remembered why they love this profession. They have hope...and every reason to believe in a future of success and joy.

My wish is that *Dynamic Dentistry* does the same for you.

—Linda Miles

WELCOME

"No employer today is independent of those about him. He cannot succeed alone, no matter how great his ability or capital. Business today is more than ever a question of cooperation."
—Orison Swett Marden, author, speaker, and founder of *SUCCESS* magazine

Ray Kroc, founder of McDonald's Corporation, was a man full of energy and driven by a powerful belief…not in burgers and fries, but in excellence. He was obsessed with quality, service, cleanliness, and value, concepts that live on today—years after his death in 1984—as the unwavering mission and identity of McDonald's.

Mr. Kroc will go down in history as the first person to create standards of quality and excellence that would one day be replicated in many thousands of McDonald's restaurants worldwide. Go to a McDonald's in London or Lisbon, and you will have largely the same experience…it will be clean, organized, and well lit. The food will taste the same, and you'll be able to order a Big Mac just the way you like it. You will feel welcomed and at home because every employee will be happy to be there, doing his or her job.

When Mr. Kroc opened his first McDonald's franchise in 1955, the concept of fast food was not new. Giants like Howard Johnson's and White Castle had been dishing up everything from burgers to thick shakes for years. Ray Kroc's genius lay in his ability to reinvent the fast food experience, using his keen understanding of what people wanted to build restaurants that required no reservations and offered low prices, no wait, and a casual environment that welcomed everyone from seniors to families with young children.

Most of all, Ray Kroc had a sense of commitment and joy about what he was doing. He was once quoted as saying, "No job on earth is insignificant if it is accomplished with pride and artistry. The french fry is my canvas. What's yours?"

Did his formula work? Of course it did. By 1963, just eight years after he opened the first McDonald's franchise, Ray Kroc had sold more than one billion hamburgers. "Spokesclown" Ronald McDonald made his debut in the same year, and by the start of the 1970s, a market researcher estimated that Ronald McDonald was familiar to ninety-six percent of American children, far more than knew the name of the president of the United States.

What on earth does all this have to do with running a dental practice?

Just about everything!

Because Mr. Kroc's is a story of success built on excellence, quality, service, and the consistent application of high standards, all concepts with tremendous power and value to the dentists and team members working in dental practices today.

It's also a story of someone who knew how to take something that had been available for many years (as dentistry has) and turn it into a fantastic success by taking a fresh, original, customer-centered approach to it…and adding his own personal passion for cleanliness and value to do it better than anyone else.

Clearly, the story of McDonald's has a great deal to teach current and future generations of business owners…small and large, in every type of business, including ours.

This is the type of thinking on which I built the concept of dynamic dentistry. That's right—*Dynamic Dentistry* is both the title of this book and an approach to practice building I've developed by working closely with several thousands of dental practices since 1978.

Starting today, I want you to begin using the proven-successful principles of *Dynamic Dentistry* to create new standards of excellence for your dental practice—ways to work faster, smarter, with more efficiency, and in a more patient-centered fashion. Day to day, month to month, and year to year, I want you to think about instituting policies and programs that will help your practice succeed and grow while ensuring that everyone associated with it wins: your coworkers, patients, suppliers, and referring dentists.

I deliberately chose the word "dynamic" to describe my approach because "dynamic" refers to energetic movement—a fast flow of ideas, information, and expertise. It's the opposite of static and unchanging. Thus, dynamic dentistry principles are specifically designed to enable your dental practice to thrive in the ever-changing business and professional environment in which it operates. That's the good news. The really good news is that once you begin, the principles of dynamic dentistry take on a life of their own, gathering a natural momentum that carries your practice forward year after year.

Ray Kroc reinvented fast food, and you and I together will reinvent the honorable, exciting, and rewarding profession of dentistry—starting with your practice. To borrow Mr. Kroc's metaphor, this is our canvas; this is our artistry.

"Begin with the End in Mind"

In his book *The Seven Habits of Highly Effective People*, professor, author, and top management consultant Steven Covey advises us to "Begin with the end in mind," by which he means that effective people structure their choices and actions around the goal or outcome they intend to achieve by the time they're through.

Dental practices around the world struggle with day-to-day operations in the areas of communication, organization, team accountability, and patient satisfaction. My goal has always been to take the mystery out of practice and team excellence while making dentistry fun, exciting, and rewarding for patients, dentists, and staff.

Dynamic Dentistry engages each and every member of a dental practice—from professionals to auxiliaries—to end this struggle by creating a practice that's built to last, in other words a profitable, well-run professional office. This concept of total professionalism, or 360 degrees of excellence as I've sometimes called it, is a main pillar of the dynamic dentistry process and one of the qualities that makes it unique.

How many times have you felt, particularly if you're a dentist or hygienist, "If all we had to do was take care of patients' teeth every day, we'd be much more successful."? If you're a business coordinator or assistant, how many times have you felt, "It would be so much easier to stay organized if these patients didn't keep interrupting me!"?

The irony is that the practice can't take care of patients unless it's done the hard work of establishing a sustainable business infrastructure in which to care for patients and ensure their satisfaction.

On the flip side, without satisfied patients, there's no need for staff or other elements of an office infrastructure!

So the goal is to improve every element of running a dental practice from patient relations to employee relations and everything in between and to establish policies and programs that continually advance the practice as a whole.

Every member of the staff must be involved and committed to this goal, and everyone must use the dynamic dentistry principles and strategies to work at it diligently every day. Experience shows that it's not the big, cataclysmic events that make or break a relationship, but rather, as Ray Kroc knew, the everyday level of excellence and quality you deliver.

Clearly, long-term success isn't just the job of the dentist as business owner. For all of us, there is a personal side to success building—it's personally contributing to service excellence in our jobs every day.

As you progress through this book, I want you to keep a few questions uppermost in your mind:

1. What do I do to deliver value to patients and to my dental practice every day?
2. What more can I do?
3. How did I deliver value today?

These are tough questions to be sure, but your answers will determine how successful both you and your practice will be.

Take a moment now to think about what inspired you to pick up this book. What information, ideas, or strategies would you like to find? What problem would you like to solve? What two or three key improvement opportunities within your practice would you like to address? Perhaps your practice is doing well in key respects, but you believe it could be doing better; there's still room for improvement.

Record your reasons on the following worksheet, assigning them a priority of high, medium, or low, as shown.

Improvement Opportunities Worksheet	
Key Problem/Opportunity	Priority [H/M/L]
1.	
2.	
3.	
4.	
5.	

Keep your goals in mind as you learn about the principles of dynamic dentistry. Refer back to this list from time to time to keep your desired outcomes at the top of your mind and to be certain that you're thinking creatively about how to apply these principles to your goals and improvement opportunities.

Get the Most Out of *Dynamic Dentistry*

Let's make a pact: in the next 205 pages, I will provide you with the tips, tactics, and techniques to be more successful than you've ever dreamed. In return, I want you to take maximum advantage of this book for yourself and your practice:

- ✧ If you have time, read the entire book once quickly, then return for a slower, more careful read. Pay particular attention to your goals and to the areas in which you feel your practice has its greatest improvement opportunities.

- ✧ Keep a separate notebook in which to record your notes, observations, your best ideas, and brainstorms to review later and share with your team.

- ✧ Underline important passages in the book, noting in particular with an asterisk concepts you believe will help you, your practice, your doctor, or your co-workers meet unique needs.

✧ Dynamic dentistry principles are comprehensive, but don't be limited by what's here. Customize the material to match your unique practice-building challenges whether they concern communication, staffing, collections, insurance, marketing, or any combination to these.

✧ Share *Dynamic Dentistry* and your notes and ideas with the others in your office in a systematic way. Devote at least half a day for the entire team to review their notes and ideas. Anticipate and prepare for the range of conversations and issues that are likely to arise.

✧ Keep *Dynamic Dentistry* handy and refer to it often. This is not a sit-on-the-shelf, once-and-done read! Dynamic dentistry principles come alive through application and implementation. Put them to work!

CHAPTER 1

Dynamic Communication: The First Step

THINK BACK TO THE SUCCESS TRIANGLE INTRODUCED EARLIER. One side represents the dentist's clinical skills, essential and irreplaceable. Another represents superior business skills that enable the practice to work efficiently, helping as many patients as possible, establishing every process and procedure needed to enable the dentist and staff to deliver superior care to as great a number of patients as possible.

The base of the Success Triangle is communication, the foundation that supports the other two, the skill upon which everything else hinges. And while great communication can't make up for poor business skills or, heaven forbid, inferior clinical skills, it can serve as the foundation that supports each of these elements, fosters key improvements, and enables them to flourish.

This is where our *Dynamic Dentistry* journey begins.

Communication Essentials

The success of any communication is the behavior it inspires. That statement usually earns me lots of blank stares in my lectures and workshops. What I mean is that communication is always aimed at motivating a certain action or set of actions. You may be trying to persuade someone to keep up the good work, pay a delinquent bill, or come in for a long-overdue preventive care appointment. Regardless, you'll only know that you've gotten through—and gotten through persuasively—by watching the person's actions afterward, noting whether they do what you want.

Communication occurs in an almost unlimited number of ways. It includes word choice, the pace of someone's speech, and tone of voice. And of course, communication isn't just verbal. A person's clothes, behavior, facial expressions, and body language all speak volumes, often before a single word is uttered.

In fact, everything we do and say communicates something, whether we want it to or not.

But there's more. Consider for instance the powerful messages sent by the appearance of your reception area and treatment rooms. Ever enter a dental practice only to see dead plants in the corner? What sort of message does that send? "You all can't even take care of a plant…How are you going to take care of my teeth?!"

Staff appearance is another important visual expression of a nonverbal message that patients hear, loud and clear. Whether they are clean and appropriate or soiled, wrinkled, provocative, or mismatched, patients are "listening" and drawing conclusions every second.

We'll consider each of these powerful communication channels as we build your practice into the dynamic, growing, and vibrant office it's meant to be.

Inside and Outside

Every business, and a dental practice is no exception, has two levels of communication dynamics: external and internal, and each is critically important to the growth and success of the practice.

External communication refers to the messages conveyed to patients and their families and to prospective patients as well. This includes the dentist and staff's interactions with them, the practice brochure and other marketing materials, even statements and recare cards. It also includes communication to insurance companies and the vendors and suppliers that support the practice. Conversations and correspondence with other dental practices whose dentists refer patients to your office and vice versa also fall into this category of communication.

External communication includes some unexpected communication channels as well: office policies, cleanliness, waiting time, and organization. These forms of "nonverbal" communication send messages about the practice's professionalism and quality, often making a more lasting impression than the written or spoken word. In fact, studies prove time and again that 80 percent of communication is nonverbal—80 percent!

Internal communication refers to everything that takes place within the practice, from casual conversations to formal staff meetings, from the structure of employee benefit programs to the appearance of the employee handbook. It's the interaction between staff members aimed at devising new strategies for ensuring patient satisfaction. It's implicit in the way the inevitable conflicts that arise in the daily press of business are handled. And it's influenced by the dentist(s) in a big way (…much more on this leadership responsibility starting on page 4).

Internal communication also includes the office environment. Is the environment in your dental office fun? Is it progressive? Is it exciting? Is it rewarding emotionally and financially? This environment does double duty as internal and external communication because of course it communicates very readily to patients as well as to staff. Patients sense when a team is happy and cohesive, and it puts them at ease. In contrast, they might feel "tension so thick you could cut it with a knife" and rightfully wonder, "Gee, maybe these guys don't really have their act together…" Their confidence and peace of mind is undermined, and the likelihood they will stay with the practice decreases dramatically.

These two communication dynamics—the internal and the external—are interdependent, which means you can't have good external communication without good internal communication, and vice versa. Yet, it's not at all unusual for an office to spend a great deal of time concentrating on the quality and frequency of its external communication while forgetting the critical importance of high quality internal communication.

Dynamic Dentistry zeros in on internal communication to start. To explain why, let me ask you a question: Would you please give me $5 million right now? Right now, cash on the barrel. No? Well, let's assume you really, really like me and you want to give me $5 million. You can't? Why not? Because chances are you don't have that kind of money hidden under your mattress. You cannot give it to me because you don't have it.

You can't give away what you don't have.

You can't communicate well externally if you're not communicating well internally.

Now, we often take it for granted that internal communication in a small dental practice is a piece of cake since everyone is right next to each other all day long. Nothing could be further from the truth! In fact, this tends to have the opposite effect: because people assume the size of the office makes communication a no-brainer, it's given short shrift causing miscommunication, unfulfilled expectations, patient attrition, and rework.

A large corporation, on the other hand, knowing it has a huge communication challenge, often an international one, makes a great effort to stay in touch with employees, shareholders, and other key audiences.

So in some ways, small businesses and professional practices must make a much more systematic effort to ensure a constant flow of information and ideas throughout the practice.

The Doctor Sets the Tone

Experience shows that—for better or worse—the "personality" of any business is a direct reflection of the personality of the individual at the helm. In a dental practice, the doctor's attitude, outlook, philosophy, and optimism level set the tone for the entire office...and often, because attitude is self-fulfilling, these personality traits determine the level of success the business achieves.

"Example is not the main thing in influencing others. It is the only thing," wrote the famous doctor and humanitarian Albert Schweitzer. This means that if you as the dentist and practice leader think your staff does a terrific job of handling patients and working as a team, you can congratulate yourself on your good leadership skills.

If, on the other hand, you cringe when you hear the way a staff member replies to a patient's question, if you overhear staff members criticizing one another, if you believe employees don't appreciate the benefits package you worked so hard to assemble for them, don't look at your staff! Look first in the mirror. Consider first the ways in which you might improve your leadership skills and the example you set.

Do you sometimes seem annoyed with patients who ask lots of questions? Do you have a tendency to harp on mistakes people make and treat disappointments as failures, rather than lessons? Have you neglected to explain the benefits package in sufficient detail to employees? Begin to take steps toward improving in these areas, and watch the positive changes that take place in your staff almost immediately.

I once worked for a dentist who exemplified the highest standards of leadership and participative management, a management tradition in which everyone's ideas were valued equally.

Dr. Wilson had a couple of immutable rules. First, if we ever heard him say or do anything that we felt was offensive to one of our co-workers or a patient, it was our job to share it with him privately. Another rule was that we were not to raise an issue or a problem without a well-considered written potential solution that could be presented for discussion at an upcoming staff meeting. Dr. Wilson encouraged us to become creative problem solvers who concentrated time and energy on devising ways to make the practice more successful.

Is it any wonder then Dr. Wilson's practice has been and will continue to be tremendously successful up until the day he retires?

Two Hours of Non-Patient Time

I am a huge fan of regular staff meetings and organizational time. In fact, I believe there is simply no way to practice dentistry in this new era of competitiveness and advancing technology without setting aside a block of non-patient time weekly to regroup as a team, tackle problems, and capitalize on new opportunities.

Yet, it's common for dentists to resist the idea of setting aside hours of non-patient time each week for organizational time. They're concerned about lost productivity, but I assure them that the practice's productivity will increase by twenty-five to fifty percent or more while everyone's stress level will decrease significantly if the team—starting with the dentist—is disciplined about having these meetings and structuring them for maximum focus and productivity.

How do you determine the optimal time of the month, week, and day to have these meetings? Simple: look at your schedule over the last three months and note the two least productive hours of each week. Chances are these fall on or about the same day each week at or about the same time of day.

This is your ideal non-patient time. You may realize for instance that the optimal non-patient time for your practice is Tuesdays from 10 a.m. to noon. Cross off this time on the schedule each week. No patient appointments may be scheduled during this time, and don't include lunch hours—no exceptions!

Structure your meetings so that weeks 1 and 3 consist of "Health of the Practice" assessments, role plays, and table clinics, and weeks 2 and 4 consist of organizational time, as follows:

Week One

In week one of each month, devote your first hour of non-patient time to a "Health of the Practice" staff meeting. During this meeting, cover practice performance data such as: What is our production per hour/day/week? What are the collections? How much are we writing off? How have these figures changed in the last month, three months, and twelve months?

Here's a list of critical performance statistics that should be covered during these meetings:

- ✧ Gross and net production (in dollars)
- ✧ Collections (in dollars)
- ✧ Collections (percentage)
- ✧ Number of new patients and emergencies
- ✧ Overhead expenses (expressed as percentage of total collections)
- ✧ The cost of supplies (expressed as a dollar figure and a percentage of total collections. The goal for dental supplies is five to seven percent.)
- ✧ The number of patients the hygienist averages per day, the number of openings in the hygiene schedule that aren't filled, and the average number of dollars produced per day by each hygienist.
- ✧ The number of patients who try to break an appointment without providing at least twenty-four hours notice

✧ Delinquent account calls made

✧ Dollars collected on bad debts

✧ The average dollars per day/hour by provider

✧ Incentive bonuses reached

✧ The number of patients who reappointed after reactivation calls as well as the number of patients who left the practice and their reasons for leaving

✧ New goals for:
- Production
- Collections
- Number of new patients

Compare the practice's current figures with historical figures, note changes, and determine the causes. Devise strategies for maximizing positive trends and stopping negative trends in their tracks.

You might compare the current figures with the prior month's figures or "this time last year" figures. If you discover that your current monthly production is up $8,500 over the same month a year ago, delve into the reasons why. What's changed? What are you doing more or less of? Why? Is this increase sustainable? For example, "We attended a perio course and hygiene increased $3,000. We had forty percent fewer broken appointments than we did in the same month a year ago."

After the "Health of the Practice" meeting, the meeting leaders should create and distribute a report of the figures reviewed and any conclusions and action plans associated with them.

Here's a useful template for creating this report:

Health of the Practice Meeting Date: ____________					
Measure	Current	One Year Ago	Increase/ Decrease	Reasons for Change	Action Steps
Gross and net production (in dollars)					
Collections (in dollars)					
Collections (as a percentage of production)					

Measure	Current	One Year Ago	Increase/ Decrease	Reasons for Change	Action Steps
Number of new patients					
Overhead expenses (expressed as a percentage of collections)					
The cost of supplies (expressed as a dollar figure and a percentage of collections)					
The number of patients the hygienist averages per day, the number of openings in the hygiene schedule that aren't filled, and/or the average number of dollars produced per day by each hygienist					
The number of patients who try to break an appointment without providing at least 24 hours notice					
Delinquent account calls made					
Dollars collected on bad debts					
The average dollars per day					
Incentive bonuses reached					

Measure	Current	One Year Ago	Increase/ Decrease	Reasons for Change	Action Steps
The number of patients who reappointed after reactination calls as well as the number of patients who left the practice and their reasons for leaving					
New goals for: -Production -Collections -New patients					

To Share or Not to Share?

Some practitioners resist the idea of sharing key office and practice statistics with employees. They fear that giving the staff information on collections, production, and expenses reveals too much about the business. However, for the most part, sharing this information is smart business because it conveys a number of essential team-building messages.

A policy of regularly sharing key practice statistics does the following:

- ✧ Demonstrates that the doctor trusts employees. (Trust breeds loyalty, reducing turnover and improving productivity over time.)

- ✧ Gives staff members clear goals and milestones to run after. (I often ask employers, "How would you like to be on a football team and play your heart out, only to never know the score?" If your staff doesn't know what's happening, how can they know what needs to happen?)

- ✧ Enables staff members to take ownership of the goals of the practice. (In this way, they avoid concluding that theirs is "just a job"—a paycheck, and nothing more.)

Over the years, I've interviewed thousands of staff members in offices where key performance statistics were not openly shared. These people almost always concluded the same thing: "My boss doesn't trust me." In more progressive (and more successful) offices, by contrast, staff members were routinely made aware of both the goals and their practices' progress toward those goals at any given point in the year. The confidentiality factor should be read before each staff meeting.

We can also look to the example set by large businesses who regularly share performance information with employees. They know that if they expect employees to take a personal interest in the success of the business, they must give them the information they need to understand the role they can play in creating that success.

If staff members are expected to think in terms of "our patients" and "our practice," they must be entrusted with statistics on the performance of the practice.

Role Plays

Reserve the second hour of non-patient time in week one for role plays. Begin gathering the information you'll need to conduct these role plays by putting a legal pad at the front desk and in every treatment room. For one solid week out of every quarter, write down every question patients ask, whether they're checking in, checking out, on the phone, or chairside. What do patients need to know? What policies, procedures, or practices confuse or trouble them? In what areas do they need more information?

Use this second hour to think through these questions by role playing and then standardize the answers patients will receive. Why is this so essential? Too often, doctors would faint if they heard some of the questions patients were asking team members...and the answers they were getting. I like to say, in addition to ensuring the accuracy of the information patients are given in response to their questions, these role plays help to ensure that every member of the team is singing from the same sheet of music. Consistency provides patients with a large measure of comfort and predictability.

Week Three

There's such power in people training people! As a result, table clinics for each department are a must. A table clinic is an opportunity to display one's talent to others. The first half hour must be delivered by the dentist(s). This is clinical dentistry 101. The second half hour is given by the hygienists. The third half hour is given by the dental assistants, and last but not least, the final half hour is given by the business staff. Below is a sample sheet of various table clinic topics each department should give on a rotation basis.

Positions	Table Clinic Topic
Assistants	✧ Inventory ✧ Lab Cases Flow System ✧ Room Set-Up and Break Down ✧ Infection Control Tips ✧ Chairside Communications ✧ Photography ✧ Materials Update ✧ Time Management (chairside) ✧ The Doctor's 10 Biggest Frustrations
Hygienists	✧ Recare System Overview ✧ Taking Radiographs ✧ Home Care Instructions ✧ The Three Stages of Perio ✧ Nutritional Counseling ✧ Setting the Stage for Case Acceptance ✧ Applying Pit and Fissure Sealants ✧ Perio Charting Terms and Explanations ✧ Use of the Intra-Oral Camera
Scheduling Coordinator	✧ The Most Frequently Asked Questions on the Phone ✧ Making an Appointment by Phone ✧ Discouraging Broken Appointments ✧ Filling Holes in the Schedule ✧ Retrieving Lost Patient Charts ✧ Greeting Procedures ✧ On-Hold Etiquette ✧ Marketing When Greeting a Patient ✧ Marketing When Dismissing a Patient

Positions	Table Clinic Topic
Office Administrator	✧ Personnel Records Management ✧ Benefits—Present and Future ✧ Practice Goals/Incentive Plan ✧ Office Policies ✧ Standard Operating Procedure Manual ✧ Team Duties—Chores ✧ Marketing ✧ The Five-Year Business Plan ✧ Staff Concerns to Doctor and Office Administrator

Weeks Two and Four

In weeks two and four of each month, use the practice's two-hour block of non-patient time for something I call organizational time. This is time you devote to the duties you can't perform in front of patients. A few examples:

- ✧ making collection calls to patients whose accounts are overdue
- ✧ following up on insurance issues
- ✧ telemarketing to "lost" patients to encourage them to return
- ✧ cleaning out the lab
- ✧ working on inventory
- ✧ editing the office policy manual
- ✧ cleaning and re-stocking each treatment area
- ✧ working on marketing plans

Whether it's hygiene, dental assisting, laboratory, or financial, each area has tasks like these that require concentrated time and no distractions. Weeks two and four become this focused, uninterrupted time. What a blessing to have time set aside every two weeks to get and stay on top of these organizational tasks and responsibilities!

Superior Staff Meetings

Frequent, well-planned staff meetings are an essential component of dynamic dentistry. Here are some tips for scheduling and running these meetings for maximum efficiency and value:

✧ Stick to the two hours week one schedule for "Health of the Practice" staff meetings and role plays. Keep this time sacred! Avoid the temptation to skip or reschedule this time; do so only for trauma emergencies.

✧ Never treat a staff meeting as a gripe session. Use the time to talk about ways to improve rather than to rehash mistakes or complain about circumstances beyond your control.

✧ Never use these meetings as a forum for criticizing individuals. Staff meetings should be a time to discuss practice problems, not people problems.

✧ Plan all staff meetings. Use an agenda focused on reviewing and discussing essential practice statistics, solving problems, and identifying areas of concern or interest to patients.

Consider giving each staff member a chance to facilitate the "Health of the Practice" staff meeting and role plays. One month the hygienist may do it, and the next someone from the business staff or an assistant or even the doctor. Rotating responsibility tends to make everyone feel equally valued and is also a great employee development tool.

You might want to set aside a portion of these meetings for progress reports presented by people representing different aspects of the practice. Each month's chosen presenter might answer the question: "What did I do last month to make the practice more successful?" Some sample areas to highlight, depending on the presenter, are:

✧ the average number of patients seen per day in hygiene

✧ the number of delinquent account calls made

✧ the number of units of C&B accepted or delivered and the comparison to the same month a year ago

This is a terrific way for everyone to enjoy the spotlight for their achievements and showcase their contributions. Staff members also become more aware of what others are doing to build the practice, thus enhancing understanding of and appreciation for the many hands and minds it takes to keep a practice humming along. Progress reports are also a great team-building tool because they help the clinical staff more fully understand the important work done by the business staff and vice versa. Progress reports also let the doctor know what has been accomplished behind the scenes in the past month, thus improving staff-to-doctor communication.

A Unique Communication Opportunity

Here's an interesting element of communication unique to dental practices: the conversation between the dentist and the assistant during treatment time. Believe it or not, this "internal" conversation is a valuable "external" communication opportunity because it has a way of distracting the patient and putting his or her mind at ease. It also conveys the rapport between the dentist and the staff and is thus a subtle but powerful marketing strategy.

Now, this conversation can be about photography, Oriental rugs, or the weather, as long as it's light, lively, and possibly educational. Dentist and staff might chat chairside about new concepts in dentistry, which communicates the staff's excitement about clinical developments as well as the practice's commitment to remain on the leading edge of modern dentistry. Discuss advances in oral hygiene or surgical advances. Talk about courses staff members have attended or plan to attend.

You should never talk about:

✧ another employee, doctor, or patient

✧ sex or politics

✧ religion

✧ upsetting topics in the news

Some patients are happy just to hear you banter about your recent ski trip. Try to include the patient in these types of conversations so they don't feel as if they're a car being worked on in the shop. You might say, "George, as soon as we take off this rubber dam, we'll let you tell us about your last ski experience, if you've had one."

This type of easy, comfortable conversation between dentist and staff sends a clear message to the patient that the practice is a strong team of people who work well together, respect one another's training and expertise, and deeply trust one another.

The doctor might further this impression by explaining, "George, Cindy's going to take over now. You're in good hands." When the doctor displays trust in the staff, the patients trust the entire practice, and the practice's loyal patient base and referrals steadily increase.

Internal Communication Has Bottom Line Value

A positive, productive working environment hinges on frequent, high quality communication between each and every member of the team. Once this caliber of communication is taking place, productivity naturally increases. Information flows easily in all directions. Guidelines are clear. Conflicts and miscommunication are minimized. Rework, that is the effort required to fix errors created by lack of communication, is a thing of the past. The practice is running on all cylinders.

Who could help but be swept up in the energy and momentum created by this exciting team of professionals working in concert toward goals they understand and believe in? Loyalty naturally increases, creating a happy working environment. Staff members begin to think in terms of what they can do for their patients and coworkers, rather than what the dentist and the practice can do for them. They work until the last patient is cared for, regardless of when their shift ends.

Patients feel more secure and refer increasing numbers of their friends and family members.

The entire practice, including every staff member and every patient, thrives on this participation, commitment, and enthusiasm. And it begins one staff member at a time. A patient coordinator working in a busy practice said it best: "I thought I needed to change jobs. But now I realize what I really needed to change was me."

Dynamic Dentistry is much more than an approach to delivering dental services efficiently and effectively. It's an exciting way to be in business with the ability to reshape the future. As a result, dynamic dentistry principles open the door to unlimited opportunities for you to have a much more direct impact on the success of the practice, and your own success too.

CHAPTER 2

Patient Communication: The Heart of Every Dynamic Dental Practice

In a very real way, patient communication is the center of every dental practice, and because of its many complexities and challenges, it demands a lot of attention and focus. The health of the office and the growth and success of the practice all depend on good quality communication between staff and patients.

In today's dental practice, the staff are valued in three ways: 1) by their clinical or business skills needed to perform their daily tasks, 2) by their team attitudes, and 3) by their ability to communicate effectively with patients, which enhances trust and boosts case acceptance.

No matter how experienced or inexperienced your dentist is, communication has the power to make or break the practice. And when problems arise or mistakes happen, communication can save the day.

External communication refers to all the ways in which messages are conveyed to patients and their families and to prospective patients as well…an enormous job, really, both in scope and in importance!

Let's start with scope. What are the elements of external communication? External communication includes:

- the dentist and staff's interactions with patients—on the phone and in person

- ✧ your practice brochure and other sales and marketing materials
- ✧ patient correspondence such as letters, statements, and recare cards
- ✧ the office's written and verbal communication to insurance companies and to the vendors and suppliers that support the practice
- ✧ the office's written and verbal communications with other dental practices whose dentists refer patients to your office and vice versa
- ✧ the practice's website

The most critical of these are the first three, and I find that the others seem to take care of themselves when the first three are well in hand.

From now on, I want you to begin acting in a way that acknowledges that everything you do and say sends a message to patients:

- ✧ Your office guidelines and policies send a message about how organized and focused you are and the practice's commitment to patients.
- ✧ The cleanliness of the office sends a message about the level of professionalism and efficiency your office delivers.
- ✧ The amount of time people spend waiting tells them how high a priority they are to the dentist and the staff members.
- ✧ The appearance of staff uniforms and nametags sends a message about the degree of professionalism and neatness of the office.

A gleaming clean office full of happy employees says, "This is a great, successful practice that every one of us is glad to be part of…and one you'll want to be part of too."

The patient coordinator's unmistakably enthusiastic greeting using the patient's name says, "We're glad to see you, and we appreciate your loyalty. We exist to provide you with excellent care and service."

If I had to sum up the purpose of this whole chapter on patient communication, it would be this: every moment of every day in every way, verbally and non-verbally, you have an opportunity to use communication as a practice-building tool. This chapter will show you how to do just that.

How would you feel if you were treated in the following manner: "Betty Johnson, follow me please"? Contrast this with: "Good morning Mrs. Johnson. My name is Debbie. I'm one of Dr. Martin's dental assistants, and we're ready for you. If you'll come right this way please…"

The first dental assistant seemed unconcerned about the comfort of the patient and treated the patient like an object or a number. The second showed a genuine customer service orientation and made the patient feel special and welcome. That's a patient who will return again and again and refer others!

Not the Place for On-the-Job Training

Chances are you're familiar with on-the-job training. Perhaps you, like me, were trained in this manner. It means that you learn on the job, usually through osmosis: by observing the actions and decisions of other more experienced team members with whom you work side by side. The idea is that you learn by examining and then repeating the skills and techniques of the person you're observing, in a kind of apprenticeship role.

On-the-job training is a way to learn from mistakes because it deliberately avoids providing the skills and information you need to sidestep these mistakes in the first place. Because a component of it is learning through trial and error—an effective and lasting learning strategy—on-the-job training can be very powerful.

I was always the last hired dental assistant, because my husband was in the Air Force for twenty-one years and we moved fourteen times. I was usually trained in this manner: "Linda just watch what we're doing here, and eventually you'll catch on."

A dental practice simply can't put an inexperienced or unskilled person on the phone with the thought, "Anybody in the world can answer the phone. How hard can it be?" And that's true of course, but there's all the difference in the world between answering a phone—a five-year-old can do that!—and answering it professionally, correctly, and helpfully. This takes maturity, in-depth training, and even a measure of skill. Like anything else, it only seems simple to the uninitiated.

Thus, in some instances, the costs of this type of training—mistakes, rework, lost patients, and lost referrals—far outweigh the advantages. Telephone technique in a dental office is clearly high on my list and should be on yours too. This is because telephone technique is a key way in which the first critical impressions are made on patients and prospective patients. When a patient is greeted on the phone in a warm and welcoming way and made to feel special, and when the person answering the phone identifies herself and uses the caller's name as soon as she knows who's calling, the patient's first impression is a strong positive one. And this first impression will last a long, long time—even through a mistake or two.

Your office must conduct regular phone role play sessions in which team members act out different parts. Videotaping a day of patient greetings and activities at the desk is a great way to identify strengths and weaknesses in the business arena. In my two-day Dental Business Conferences held throughout the U.S., Canada, New Zealand, and Australia, we deliberately demonstrate poor examples of telephone skills in order to contrast these with the best examples taken from the most successful practices we know.

For example: some busy business staff members have managed to convince their doctors that the phone keeps them from other important duties. The result is that the phone is answered electronically instead of by a person. This works in some businesses quite well; dental practices—personal and private by their very nature—are not among them. In fact, we consider it the kiss of death for any dental practice to have voice mail taking calls during patient hours. In dynamic dental practices, a human being answers the phone during business hours...period.

Image Is Everything

I recently added a division to my business called "Image Is Everything." This recognizes that people want to do business with people they perceive as professional. The reason that image is everything is that perception is everything and the image of the office and the staff creates an instant perception in the patient's mind. The practice can send a visual image that conveys competence and cleanliness or one that communicates something less...all through the power of perception. If you go to the bank and there are five tellers, none of whom are occupied, chances are you'll do a quick visual survey and go to teller who looks the most professional.

We determined there was a strong need for this type of service because we saw over the years such a wide spectrum of "business" dress in dental practices around the country: everything from "Betty the Banker" dressed in pinstripes and sporting a severe hairstyle to "Super-Casual Cathy" in stretch stirrup pants and a long T-shirt. I've even seen go-go boots and mini-skirts!

The "Image Is Everything" process begins with the creation of office guidelines for appropriate attire for the practice. These should be clear, complete, and given to each new employee before they begin work, if possible. The key question to answer in these guidelines is, "What type of image are we trying to project?"

Office Image

If a practitioner wants upscale clients, he or she must present an upscale office image. Patients and people in general like to "shop up," meaning we prefer to associate with services and suppliers that are as upscale as possible, within our budget limitations. When we select a restaurant, supermarket, retail store, car dealership, or vacation spot, we shop on the high end, even though we all look for bargains from time to time and love to tell about how much we saved.

When it comes to health care in general and dentistry in particular, patients may complain about the fees, but they select the practitioner who will do their dentistry by the office, dentist, and staff images. Some patients may even go as far as to ask you if they're paying for the upscale office with the veneers they just had placed or the bridge they need.

To help prevent these sorts of questions, when one of my clients builds a new office or invests in a significant upgrade to their present facility, I recommend placing a sign at the front desk that reads, "Our office has recently been fully rebuilt (redecorated) in appreciation of our wonderful patients." When patients realize the upgrade was completed in their interest, they're much more appreciative and less likely to think or say, "I guess I'm paying for all this!"

Years ago, I was privileged to hear one of dentistry's pioneer speakers, Dr. Ken Olsen, say, "When a patient complains about their fee or says, 'I guess

I'm paying for this,' the dentist, staff members, or spouse of the dentist should nicely pull out a small note pad from their pocket, drawer, or purse and say, 'Let me see now...you're Mrs. Freeman. No, according to my records, Mr. Jones paid for that chair, but you paid for our trip to Hawaii. Thank you SO MUCH!'" If you feel comfortable, it's perfectly appropriate to use humor to diffuse the situation, and get the patient to laugh with you.

It's impossible to overemphasize the need to keep the office appearance neat and organized. How disheartening it is for patients to see a dentist spend hundreds of thousands of dollars to provide a beautiful office that ends up cluttered and messy. While I hope every practice has a cleaning service to clean the floors, plumbing fixtures, and empty the trash, it is truly the total team's responsibility to keep the office spotless and uncluttered during the working day and have it totally presentable for patients every hour of the day. Each dental team member should have an area within the office that he or she must keep clean and organized throughout the day.

Doctor's Image

The doctor's image is as important, if not more so, than the work environment—the physical office itself—for attracting a certain type of clientele. The vast majority of patients will choose dentists who make them feel comfortable by dressing the way they do.

The dentist should dress casually (golf shirts for men, cotton blouses for women, khaki pants, and casual shoes) to attract a mid-tier clientele. To attract white-collar professionals, the dentist must wear dress slacks, dress shirts, and nice executive shoes...like a business professional, but on a more comfortable level (with lab coats for OSHA regulations).

Business Staff Image

Dentistry is a health care profession, which means cleanliness and neatness in professional appearance are paramount. Some practices provide staff uniforms; thus, image tends to be a non issue. The image of these offices is total uniformity and it has its advantages. From the patient's perspective, these offices look fairly well pulled together.

For this reason, I highly recommend that the office provide a uniform allowance for all staff so they can dress in coordinating professional fashion. Most offices provide scrubs or uniforms for clinical staff. Some of my clients buy pieces of clothing like the airlines and permit the business staff to mix and match these pieces for a uniform yet individual look.

I have always felt that business staff should wear business attire, not clinical attire. Choose inexpensive blazers and blouses or vests and blouses, plus slacks or skirts that coordinate with the office colors (try picking up on the colors in the rug or on the walls or window treatments) and the clinical staff's scrubs. This sends a strong message about the cohesiveness of the team. It also ensures that the staff's dress or accessories will not distract the patient in any way. Staff should be dressed professionally and in an understated fashion that makes clothes a non issue, not a distraction to patients.

Some additional guidelines:

- ✧ Socks and shoes are not appropriate at the front desk. Women should choose flats or low heels and stockings instead.
- ✧ Every staff member must wear a nametag, because within two minutes of hearing your name, patients have already forgotten it.
- ✧ Make-up should be used moderately and be in good taste for a health care practice: no vivid eye shadows or black nail polish, for instance.
- ✧ Avoid wearing fragrance; however, if you choose to wear perfume or cologne, be certain it has a light fragrance and apply it very sparingly.
- ✧ There should be clear guidelines on body piercing and tattoos.

Some dentists have sent their team members on a fun outing to a professional makeover at a department store or home party. Throwing in a gift certificate to start employees on the path to an improved self-image can be highly motivating and helpful to the team.

Clinical Team Image

All dental assistants and hygienists must look the part of a well-groomed clinical employee in every sense. Scrubs must be pressed rather than look like wrinkled pajamas. Shoes should be scrubbed, sprayed, polished, buffed...whatever it takes to make them bright and clean. Believe it or not, patients judge the cleanliness of the instruments by the cleanliness of the clinical staff shoes.

Tennis shoes are acceptable as long as they are spotless and not a pair that the employee wears to mountain climb or mow the grass in on the weekends. In fact, if the dentist and staff have small children crawling around on the floors at home, for infection control measures, I highly recommend leaving clinical shoes at the back door of the office in shoe cubicles and not wearing them on the carpets of their vehicles or at home.

It's been my professional experience and that of my clients that when we look our worst, we feel our worst. Even on days when I'm not 100 percent, if I spend fifteen minutes using my best effort to fix my hair and cover my flaws, I feel 100 percent better when I meet the public or myself if I pass my reflection in a mirror! And it never fails, on days I skip my routine, I run into everyone I know or neighbors I rarely see drop over for no particular reason. Though I've been working at home since the summer of 2000, I still get ready as if I'm meeting my most important client even if I'm in casual clothes and may only see my husband and the UPS delivery person. Being well groomed, no matter what, is of great importance.

The Practice's Image on Paper

Start by looking at every piece of paper you hand out or mail from your office. If it does not reflect the image you are trying to project, it is time to hire a professional graphic artist or marketing company to assist with this very important part of the image mix. You and your dentistry are a direct reflection of the image on paper that your office displays.

If you don't have a logo, have one created for your practice (see page 180), and keep in mind that a happy tooth dancing around outside a mouth is outdated and too playful for today's world of dentistry. Messages like "gentle dental" and "We cater to cowards" are also a bit passé.

For much more on managing every aspect of your image, read *Image Matters, First Steps on the Journey to Your Best Self*, by Lauren Solomon

(Education/Exposure Publications, New York, 2002); available through LLM&A at www.dentalmanagementU.com. Lauren, whose company Strategic I Image Consulting helps individuals and businesses improve their image from the inside out and outside in, has a powerful saying: "Cultivate your image deliberately and strategically, and all doors will open before you." This is how important image is to practice success…and to individual success as well.

The Eight Phases of Patient Communication

Dynamic dentistry is built on eight phases of patient communication. I refer to these as "phases" because patient communication moves through a process from the initial impression on the phone through the entire visit to the last impression as the patient exits the practice.

Each patient has different information needs at different times of their visit. Considering each phase individually will help you keep this flow in mind. At any given point in the day, each team member will be communicating with different patients at different phases of their visits. Thinking in terms of phases of patient communication also enables you to keep in mind that each phase offers a unique opportunity to make a positive impression on a given patient.

Before I launch into a scientific-sounding discussion of dynamic dentistry's strategy for ensuring practice-building patient communication, I want to underscore a few simple facts about communication. First, remember that communication is an exchange of ideas and information that takes place between two people. One speaks; one listens. There is understanding and action as a result. My main point is that if we set our starting point at sincerely trying to make a connection to another person to impart information in a way that will genuinely help that person, a great deal of the dynamic dentistry communication phases and principles fall naturally in place.

Second, good communication with patients is based on respect and gratitude…respect for each patient as unique and gratitude that a patient chose your practice over the many others available.

Good patient communication also saves time and increases productivity. Staff members skilled in good communication save their dentists many hours a week, freeing up the dentist's time to concentrate more fully on clinical dentistry, which of course positively impacts revenue and profit levels for the practice.

So it's absolutely not a coincidence that the most successful practices—and I've seen and helped to create thousands of them—are filled with smiling, pleasant employees skilled at communicating effectively with patients at all phases of the patient's visit.

A New Title

Although every member of the dental team is equally important, the person at the front desk interacts with patients in five out of the eight phases of patient communication, compared with three for the assistant or hygienist and one for the doctor. Therefore, most of the responsibility for practice building through good communication skills rests with the person or employees at the front desk.

One of the very first things I ask every client to do is dispense with the word "receptionist" in referring to this person. The person who sits at the front desk must greet patients warmly by name, answer the phones, and engineer the schedule and the office workflow. This is a job of critical importance to the health, growth, and profitability of the practice. This person is also the practice's unofficial public relations agent. She determines a patient's first and last impression of the practice.

Why in the world would you put a title like "receptionist" on someone with this much influence on practice building? The title doesn't match the job; it's so much more than simply receiving people, as the title receptionist implies.

Replace the word "receptionist" with patient care facilitator, business coordinator, or scheduling coordinator. Now there's a title that aptly reflects the integral role this person plays in the daily, profitable operation of the office.

A Word about Tone

It's not what we say; it's how we say it that matters most. Ten different people might say the same phrase and give it different meaning just through their tone of voice. Think of the number of ways you might hear the simple phrase, "Thank you." It can be said with enthusiasm, sarcasm, frustration, high or low energy, a smile, a frown, or in monotone, with no expression at all. Each tone of voice enables the very same words to send distinctly different messages.

Dynamic dentistry's practice-building patient communications begin with the realization that tone of voice alone can send the message that your practice is friendly, staff members are knowledgeable and excited, and that you have the empathy and concern essential for working in a care-giving field.

Tone is so important that I tell clients if the person answering your phone does not come across as well as they should, it is killing your practice before it has a chance to grow. And here's the really scary part: the dentist/owner won't even know. These patients will silently do something I call "voting with their feet." They'll choose another practice that makes them feel comfortable, with a staff whose tone makes it seem as if they're genuinely glad to be there...and they'll never say a word to you about it.

There are four aspects of your tone of voice that help to build a healthy, growing practice. I call these aspects of tone your "must haves." Your tone must be:

1. friendly
2. knowledgeable
3. enthusiastic
4. empathetic

Let's take these aspects one by one. Number one is friendly. If your practice isn't a friendly place, you'll have a lot of hang-ups and "I'll call you backs." We've all had the experience of calling an office—whether it was the local shoe retailer, an insurance agent, or a widget company—and hearing the person answering the phone say, "[Name of company]. Can you hold?" You don't even get the chance to say "Okay" before you hear a click and land in the silent or Muzak-filled netherworld of "hold"! This is distinctly "unfriendly" treatment of that business's greatest asset: its customers. (Never put someone on hold until you know who it is and ask permission!)

In your efforts to be friendly, remember that every person in the world has a sign on their forehead that says, "Make me feel important." How many times have you had reservations at a nice restaurant and walked up to the person who will seat you and your guests, only to have them say, "Do you have a reservation?" Not "Welcome to Such-and-Such restaurant," but the equivalent of, "Do we even know who you are?" Then, perhaps something like, "Well, I don't see your name here. What did you say your name was? Duncan? Dumont?"

"Um, no, Davis," you reply.

They don't make you feel special, and regardless of how good the food is, you probably won't return.

On the flip side, have you ever walked into a restaurant with friends you're trying to impress, perhaps company from out of town or even a business acquaintance, and the maitre d' says, "Dr. Davis, your table is waiting. I made it your special table." Now, the food could be mediocre, but you'll go back because the service was so good. No question that friendliness and making people feel special and important enter into the practice-building picture big time. They are absolutely essential to practice building.

Second, each team member must be knowledgeable. Can everyone on your team—whether they've been with the practice thirteen years or three months—answer basic questions about dentistry, the doctor, and his or her practice, questions like:

- ✧ "How long has the dentist been practicing?"
- ✧ "What dental school did he or she graduate from?"
- ✧ "Do you use the latest technology?"
- ✧ "Does the dentist perform oral surgery?"
- ✧ "How often should I have my teeth cleaned?"
- ✧ "Are x-rays safe?"

Does each staff member know how to respond to patient concerns that go beyond simple fact-based questions? Concerns like:

- ✧ "I am so nervous. I've always been terrified of dentists."
- ✧ "I've neglected my mouth for ten years, and I'm very embarrassed now to go to a dentist, but I have to go in because I have a problem."
- ✧ "The last dentist I went to worked on this tooth, and now it's worse."

If a patient says, "I'm so nervous. I've always been terrified of dentists," people who practice dynamic dentistry principles know never to gloss over this fear but rather to acknowledge it by saying something like, "Well, you know Mrs. Jones, you have called the right office, because we specialize in patients who have felt apprehensive in the past, and they are our greatest referral sources today." This reply gives the patient confidence and helps calm her down.

Why is a knowledgeable tone so important? The most important reason is that it conveys confidence and composure, which communicates very readily to patients. As if by osmosis, they begin to feel confident and composed. They believe they've called the right office, and they'll be treated with the utmost care, concern, expertise, and professionalism.

Third on my list of "must haves" is enthusiasm. What does enthusiasm in someone's voice communicate to the patient? That's obvious: it says, "I love my job, and I am delighted to help you." Again, another powerful confidence booster for patients. A contented employee is likely to do a better job, and to patients, a better job means high quality dental care and adept handling of all the details that precede and follow that care.

An enthusiastic tone has a smile and a nice, light pace to it. Even when you're very, very busy, I want you to answer the phone with, "Thank you for calling Dr. Martin's office. This is Linda. How may I help you?" Notice, I didn't say, "May I help you" but rather "How may I help you?" There's all the difference in the world between the two. "How may I help you" is active and asks the patient what he needs right away, and has the implicit message that "I can help you because I'm trained and competent in how to help you." The idea is of course that everyone calling needs help from you, so asking how you can supply that help is good business.

Helpful Hint

My friend and colleague Joy Millis suggests that, though an enthusiastic greeting is essential, dental offices should avoid answering the phone with "Good morning" or "Good afternoon" because in a busy practice, it's impossible to know whether it's morning or afternoon. If you're in an office that's windowless, you really have a problem knowing morning from afternoon. So instead of "Good morning" or "Good afternoon," simply thank the caller for contacting the office, provide the doctor's name, and ask how you can help.

Finally, your tone must convey *empathy*, a quality essential in any caregiving profession. Every dentist and every dental staff member should have an excruciating toothache at least once in their lives so they'll have empathy for an emergency. Empathy is the quality of putting yourself in the patient's shoes, and it is absolutely essential for any dental practice, not only for the people who arrive in pain, but for those who are embarrassed about having neglected their teeth, those who are having difficulty paying, and those who have two crying children with them while they're trying to have their teeth cleaned.

The Phases One by One

The dynamic dentistry model organizes patient communication into eight phases. I do this for a variety of reasons. It's easy to think about communication in separate phases. It makes certain you don't miss anything. At each phase in the patient's visit, the patient's emotional and information needs are different and so it helps to look at each one separately. At any given point in your day, patients will be at different stages of their visits, and knowing how to handle each one will help you to handle multiple priorities such as patients and computers at the same time.

The eight phases occur throughout a patient's visit. A full seven of the eight are interactions solely between the patient and staff members. Once again, it's clear that good communication skills on the part of staff members are essential in practice building.

Phase One: Telephone

Answering the telephone is the most important phase of all communication. A person's first—and often most lasting—impression of a dental office is formed in the first thirty seconds of telephone contact. You may never get a second chance to correct a "Hello" that was grumpy. However, a caller can receive an instant impression of a happy, caring doctor's office if the person answering has a smile in their voice.

This cheerfulness on the phone has a serendipitous side effect: patients who are sitting in the reception area are reassured and cheered by the sound of a pleasant voice.

Successful practices will get 300 to 400 new patients a year per doctor, or thirty-three per month. That is a lot of "first impressions" to make, which means that the phone is a powerful marketing tool…if it's used well. When patients are made to feel important on the phone, the entire tone of the dental experience gets off to a great start.

Investing in more telephone lines and learning to use them repays itself many times over. Answering the telephone in a cheerful and caring manner makes every patient feel special.

Voice mail is wonderful in some companies, but I don't think it's wonderful in dentistry. No matter how busy and large your practice gets, a human being must answer your telephone during office hours…even, if possible, during lunch hours. I sincerely hope that if you have a phone system that goes to voice mail during office hours, you will change that because we're not selling widgets or insurance. Dentistry is a care-giving, people-oriented business.

Here are some strategies for maximizing the practice-building value of the telephone in your office:

✧ Answer on the first few rings.

If the scheduling coordinator cannot answer the telephone on the first few rings, the office is understaffed. This is a problem in many dental practices. Patients calling the office can only hear the ringing or busy signal. They cannot see a patient standing in front of the desk, being helped. However, the patient at the desk hears the telephone and understands that it must be answered.

✧ No busy signals!

When new patients get busy signals, they may forget to call back, or, worse yet, look for another dentist who isn't so busy. A busy signal is one of the fastest ways to kill a dental practice. Putting a patient on hold is also a quick way to chill enthusiasm. Being placed on hold says very clearly that the caller is not important enough to rate immediate attention. Subsequent efforts to sound happy and caring tend to be dismissed by those who have been on hold too long.

The person answering the phone may have top notch telephone skills, but she won't have an opportunity to use these skills properly if the practice has only one incoming phone line.

Remember, busy people hate busy signals. An investment in adequate equipment is insignificant compared to the new patients who may be lost by an office appearing to be too busy. A dental practice can only be as adequate as the telephone system.

✧ Handle multiple calls deftly.

Most dental offices should have no less than two incoming lines and a third private line for outgoing calls and occasional incoming personal calls. A competent scheduling coordinator will be able to handle three lines in a professional manner. The first caller always has priority, so make the second answer brief…call back if you must. Never answer with, "Can you hold please?" Click. To the first caller say, "Excuse me, Mrs. Holmes, my other line is ringing. I'll be back in less than sixty seconds." Put the call on hold; pick up the second line and say, "Thank you for calling Dr. Wood's office. This is Mary. I'm on another call. Will you hold for a few moments or may I call you back?" And remember, anytime anyone is on hold, brevity is key. A full minute on hold feels like an eternity to the person holding. Information on hold is a great marketing tool that provides patient education about dentistry, the practice, and doctor(s). There are message on hold messenging companies available, but I prefer Patient Pro. Their toll-free number is 866-865-4055.

✧ Identify yourself.

Always answer the phone by identifying yourself and the office. If you identify the office only, the caller is speaking with an object. By identifying yourself, you've begun on a friendly, caring note with the caller. It's annoying for a caller to have to ask, "Is this Betty, Joan, or Mary?" Even in a one business staff member office, it is still good telephone manners for the answering person to identify herself.

Here are two examples of how NOT to answer the phone:

Example 1:

"Dr. Martin's office. Can you hold please?"

This call seems to be an interruption of the scheduling coordinator's busy day.

Example 2:

"Dr. Martin's office ...yes....uh, I'm really not sure; I can ask the hygienist. Can you hold for a moment please?"

When the employee doesn't identify herself, the caller is talking to an "office."

Here's what your phone greeting should sound like: "Thank you for calling Dr. Martin's office. This is Linda. How may I help you?...Yes, Mr. Fairlin. Your appointment is tomorrow at 10:00 a.m., and we're looking forward to seeing you then. Thank you for calling."

The ideal telephone etiquette enables patients to feel that they are being treated with care and concern. The office is clearly identified, and the person answering the telephone is friendly and wants to know that patient.

✧ Avoid this classic mistake:

One of the biggest telephone mistakes in a dental office is asking the caller, "Have you been a patient here before?" Even if the person answering the phone is new to the practice, there is the risk of insulting patients of record by failing to recognize them. People love to feel important. The caller may be someone who completed a large treatment plan last month. If you don't know the caller, ask, "How long has it been since your last appointment with the doctor?" This strategy eliminates the risk of insulting either a new or former patient.

✧ If the caller is a new patient:

If the caller is a new patient, the scheduling coordinator answering the phone must find out whether the person needs a routine office visit or help with a particular problem by asking, "Are you having an immediate problem, Mrs. Jones?"

Avoid words like "pain" or "hurt" because they are negative words (see Appendix A). If the new patient indicates they're having an immediate problem, the staff should be maximally responsive. Emergency patients become enthusiastic missionaries for dental practices. (See Chapter 6 for much more on emergencies.)

✧ Limit personal calls.

Everyone knows that excessive personal calls disrupt the workflow and efficiency of any office. The patient coordinator who spends a lot of time answering calls for the doctor and staff about their personal business is distracted, harried, and unable to do other productive, practice-building work.

And, more to the point, anything that unnecessarily shortchanges patients of the team's undivided attention should be scrutinized carefully and addressed as quickly as possible.

Phase Two: Greeting/Welcome

Sometimes the only difference between one dental office and another is how the patient is welcomed and put at ease. Think about that for a moment. Every patient who enters a dental office is at least a little apprehensive. As a result, one of the key responsibilities of front desk personnel is to make patients feel at ease.

People at the front desk must be aware of the names on the appointment schedule and greet patients by name when they arrive. As each patient enters, the person at the front desk may say something like, "Good morning; you must be Mr. Black. My name is Susan. I spoke with you on the phone yesterday," never, "Have a seat; I'll be with you in a moment."

When a patient enters a dental practice, he or she should feel very special, like a guest in someone's home. If you were to walk into a dental office in which everyone seemed preoccupied and didn't treat you well, chances are you wouldn't come back.

Example 1

"I'll be with you in a moment."

The patient certainly isn't greeted warmly, and it's obvious that the scheduling coordinator is busy and couldn't really look up to acknowledge the patient other than to say a few emotionless words.

Example 2

"Do you have an appointment today?"

Clearly, there's some confusion about whether this patient should even be in the office.

Example 3

"Yes, and I would like to make an appointment to have my hair colored and

cut. Yes, just a trim, and...I'll be with you in a moment. Yes, have anything on a Friday afternoon, I'm off on Friday afternoon. Oh, I don't think that day will work, I think we're going out of town that weekend, let me think, probably the seventh would be better. Okay. It will be with Carol. Thank you so much. Um, may I help you?"

One of the worse things that can happen with patient welcoming is that the staff person is tending to personal business at the front desk. There should never be anything more important than the patient who's actually paying everyone's paycheck.

Example 4

"Good morning! You must be Mrs. Johnson. My name is Linda. I spoke with you on the phone yesterday. Welcome to Dr. Martin's practice."

The welcome in a dental practice is very important, not only to existing patients but also to new patients. When a new patient enters the reception area, I hope that you stand, smile, extend your hand, and introduce yourself. In doing so, you convey to the patient that he or she is important to you, which is precisely what an introduction is designed to do in the first place!

There is no sweeter sound to a person than that of his own name. When you use it, you instantly endear the person to you and build rapport in a moment's time. Staff members should get in the habit of addressing patients by name during conversation. If the scheduling coordinator is too busy to give a warm, friendly greeting, the office is either understaffed or the scheduling coordinator is not the right "people person" to have at the front desk. A warm, expressive person at the front desk is vital to practice building.

Make the patient feel that he or she is the most important person to walk through the office door that day. Highlight new patient names in the appointment scheduler for easier recognition and a special welcome.

Open or Closed?

Take a moment one day in the near future to walk outside your dental practice and walk in as a patient would. What do you see? How are you greeted? Hopefully not with the little movie theater window that slides open to reveal someone's face.

I think the open concept is the only way to go with business staff. There are several reasons why I like there to be no wall and no window, simply a wraparound countertop as the front desk:

1. In an open environment, you're "on stage" and more professional. When you have walls and windows to hide behind, you can bring your coffee, toast your muffin under the desk, and eat M&M's out of your desk drawer. None of these is possible when the front desk is an open countertop. (It's okay to have a glass of water, or maybe a coffee, as long as it can't spill all over the computer.)

2. It's friendlier since there's no real barrier between you and your patients sitting in the reception area, many of them for the very first time.

3. The doctor and clinical staff cannot come up and visit and disrupt workflow when they're not busy. In some practices the clinical team and doctor congregate at the desk when they are not busy. This is a distracting habit that wastes valuable time that should be devoted to patient care.

Phase Three: Registration

The third phase, registration, is often perceived as a dry, fill-out-this-form part of the patient's visit. But it can be much more than that. Like all phases of patient communication, registration can be a valuable marketing and sales opportunity.

Registering a patient is a simple procedure. Some offices like to "romance" patients by filling out the forms for them. In most offices, however, patients are asked to fill out their own registration and health histories while waiting for their appointments. Generally, a patient would rather write the information than have to say aloud that he or she is unemployed, has a bladder problem, or hasn't seen a dentist for eight years.

Occasionally patients may forget their glasses or need help for other reasons. Don't wait for them to ask for help. Offer assistance by saying, "Please fill out this information sheet, front and back, and pay particular attention to the health questions. Dr. Wood is interested in your total health. I'll be glad to help, if you like."

Example 1:

"Hi, Mrs. Johnson. I'll need you to fill out some patient information. Help yourself to the clipboard, and when you're finished, just bring it back to me."

In registering the patient, the last thing you want to do is make it look like a do-it-yourself office. You'll notice in this example that the scheduling coordinator was too preoccupied to even stand, much less give the patient complete instructions.

Example 2:
"Mrs. Johnson, this is a very important patient registration form. We're interested in any employee benefit coverage that you may have, and also your medical history. When you finish side one, please turn it over and continue. If you have any questions or you need any help, I'm here to assist you."

> **Important!**
> *The first three phases of communication (telephone, greeting, and registration) take a total of about ten minutes. In this brief time, patients have decided whether they like being part of the practice and whether they will refer their family and friends to you. Keep the critical importance of this time in your mind as we move on.*

Phase Four: Seating the Patient/Pretreatment Education
Have you had the experience of waiting in a physician's office sometimes as long as two hours? You're just about to leave in total frustration when a staff member finally comes into the reception area and says, "Mrs. Jones?"

You stand up and follow the person trance-like into a cold little room. It's pretty sparse, with a table covered in white crunchy paper. You're told to undress and put on a gown with some unspeakable opening that goes in the front or the back, depending on what you're there for. They take your clothes and tell you the doctor will be with you shortly, which ends up being another forty-five minutes sitting on the cold paper in the humiliating gown, with nothing to read. Now that they've taken your clothes, you cannot leave. So you sit basically naked in your sensory deprivation tank, waiting, waiting.

Keep this scene in mind as you consider my rule of thumb for patient seating in a dynamic dental practice: never seat until you are ready to treat. Do not escort the patient to the treatment room and force them to sit and wait nervously—every patient is at least a bit apprehensive, no matter how unaffected they may try to appear.

Now, I'm well aware that many times the dentist urges staff, "Get them back there. Just get them back there!" in the interest of keeping the patient flow going. And while there's some value in smooth patient flow, be certain you're not forcing patients to sit alone in a cold room, nervous, with nothing to read and no one to talk to.

After patients are seated, they should never be left without a word of explanation. If they are seated and left alone, they wonder what is going on. Fear and apprehension are real and tend to be magnified by the unknown. If you must leave the room, explain when you'll return. Be certain that every treatment room has magazines suitable for men, women, and children, as well as patient education materials

Use the time after seating the patient to:

- ✧ Explain that nearly every patient has some degree of apprehension about a dental treatment. Fear in patients is normal, and all patients need to know they are not alone in feeling apprehensive.
- ✧ Conduct some dental education. This may include a pre-treatment explanation like, "Mrs. Miles, today we're going to be doing thus and so." Describe the procedure and talk about the patient's immediate-term and long-term experience and the wisdom in making an investment in this procedure.
- ✧ Praise the patient's decision to have whatever procedure they are sitting in the chair for.
- ✧ Convey your enthusiasm for the dental profession, for working with people in a care-giving role, and for your particular practice: "I work for the greatest dentist in the whole world" or "I probably have the best job in this town. I love what I do."

Many dental auxiliaries don't "talk dentistry." In my experience, this usually happens for two reasons: First, they don't have the time. They're too harried with patient and nonpatient duties to stop and talk to a patient, much less deliver information that takes time and concentration to impart. (This is a staffing problem I'll tackle later in Chapter 4.)

Second, the dentist has never delegated these conversations to staff or trained the staff to have these conversations with patients…a common mistake and a lost opportunity to increase practice productivity. More on this later too.

Begin by wearing a smile that radiates warmth and enthusiasm, no matter how difficult your day has been or how long it's been since you've taken a coffee break. Patients have no idea of these things, nor do they care. Their only concern—and yours too—should be their treatment.

This type of handling during the pretreatment phase accomplishes a few things: it enables patients to know who you are and what you do. Your air of calm poise communicates that you're in control of the situation and that you do this all the time. Your confidence means to them that you also have confidence in the doctor, in the quality of patient care being delivered. All these factors instill trust and reduce patients' fears.

It also gives patients a clear sense that you like the doctor and the practice, with the subtle suggestion that they should too. It's extremely unsettling to be helped by someone you don't know, whose name you don't know, whose role you don't know. You feel like an object.

A patient might ask you quietly, "Do you like working here?" or "Why did the last assistant leave?" Patients ask such questions because their confidence in the office is related to how well the staff members and the doctor like each other.

If a patient asks, "Do you like working here?" answer with, "I enjoy it very much. I like working with people and this is a great team. We're serious when we need to be, but we also have fun."

If a patient asks, "Why did the last assistant leave?" answer with, "You know, I'm not one-hundred percent sure, but I think she wanted to pursue another opportunity. We all wish her the best. She did a great job, and we'll miss her."

(Of course, if the reason is a positive one, such as a marriage that required the assistant to relocate with a new spouse or a decision to stay home full-time with a new baby, feel free to share the good news with the patient. The goal is to convey as positive a message as possible.)

I once heard about a dental assistant who would seat patients without so much as looking at them. She was once observed going into the reception area with a patient's chart in her hand. One woman and two men were waiting and she looked up without acknowledging who was there and said, "Which one of you is Florence?" I'd have paid money to see one of the men joke, "I am!"

Phase Five: Treatment

The doctor must always be aware of the patient's name and the reason for the visit. This information should be available on the daily work list that is present in each treatment room or on the computer screen if the office is paperless.

During treatment time, the chairside assistant should show concern for and interest in the patient. It's frustrating to the doctor if the assistant is preoccupied with unimportant things, looks at her watch frequently, or daydreams. Dental assisting can become repetitive, but there is a patient attached to every tooth you treat. Patients always deserve full attention and nothing less.

Conversation is acceptable during treatment as long as it does not exclude or frustrate the patient because of his or her inability to join in. Small talk can be effective to relieve anxiety, but much depends on the doctor's and patient's personalities as well as the situation. The doctor and staff should never discuss personal problems in the presence of patients. Light personal conversation such as "How was your vacation?" or "I saw your daughter's wedding picture in the paper," helps build rapport. Never discuss personal problems that are "downers." In one office an assistant burdened every patient with the minute details of her divorce. Most folks have enough problems of their own and don't need to hear someone else's. And never—ever—discuss religion or politics...these are generally hot topics on which people often disagree.

Phase Six: Patient Education

Why would I devote an entire phase of communication to patient education? Because in a dynamic dental practice, patients are in an active partnership with the dentist and the entire dental practice team. Indeed, a healthy mouth requires a partnership between patient and dental office because the office can only do so much. The rest is up to the patient's commitment to daily oral hygiene at home.

Patient education is good business too. Dentists who train their assistants and hygienists in how to educate patients as a rule have higher production than those who don't. It makes sense: The dentist's time is freed up to treat other patients. In addition, by turning patients over to clinical staff members, doctors ensure that rapport is built with the entire staff, not just with themselves. Patients also have greater confidence in the expertise of the entire office; everyone knows what they're doing and can be relied on for information and expert help. Patients are also often more comfortable asking the assistant questions that they won't ask the doctor, either out of general discomfort or intimidation or because they perceive they're wasting the doctor's time.

Dentists with the greatest skill in this area have mastered the art of smoothly turning the patient over to the appropriate staff member. The key to patient acceptance in this phase is for doctors to verbalize their trust by saying, "Ms. Johnson, it was nice seeing you. I look forward to your next visit. Sherry will be spending time with you now." The doctor can then be five to ten minutes into another procedure while being assured that Ms. Johnson is receiving first-class information and patient education from Sherry.

Sherry might then explain, "Mrs. Johnson, today the doctor restored six surfaces of those two teeth. You may experience a slight discomfort when you eat or drink something cold. Some of our patients experience this, but others never do. If this happens it's perfectly normal. It could last a week or two. Mrs. Johnson, we don't expect any problems with this procedure, but if you have any questions after you leave, here is my personal business card. Please call me." Notice, she doesn't say, "If you have any problems, call me." Such a statement plants negative seeds and encourages problem calls. Ironically, patients never call staff at home but the thought that they would be available for an emergency call is a great practice builder.

The assistant should also review postoperative instructions and provide written instructions for extractions, periodontal surgery, and endodontic treatments. In some instances, families of patients need written information for proper home care.

Before dismissing a patient, the assistant should say, "Before you leave, Ms. Hall, are there any questions you'd like to ask?" Don't be concerned that the patient will ask you a question you either can't answer or don't feel comfortable answering. If this happens, simply say, "Ms. Hall, I feel Dr. Wood should answer that question. He's with another patient at the moment. May I take a telephone number where you can be reached during the next hour? I will call you with his answer."

After all questions are answered, the assistant or hygienist should walk patients to the front desk, hand the patient her chart, and say, "Please give your chart to Mary at the front desk so she can give you your receipt for today's visit" or "Please give your chart to Mary at the front desk so she can process your insurance immediately so that you may file it for immediate reimbursement"...and we move on to Phase Seven.

Phase Seven: Reappoint and Present Fee

Let me begin Phase Seven with the hope that every dental practice is using computer care slips. If you are not using computer-generated care slips, you're hurting the communication flow from the front desk to the treatment rooms and back again.

Computer care slips serve two important purposes. They are your only communication from the back office to the front office, and they are your only internal audit to ensure that every procedure performed on a given day goes into the accounting system. Have your financial coordinator total your care slips daily, and you have a superior internal audit tool. The computer care slips must match the clinical record on all x-rays, sealants, and other procedures. Many dental practices could go around the world three times on the money lost on mistakes that are unintentionally made in the posting of treatments performed each month. If you have computer terminals chairside, care slips are still a must-have for the internal audit daily.

Chairside Terminals

With the advent of chairside terminals, the entire focus of patient flow is changing. I'm very excited about the clinical team being able to enter the treatment just performed and make the next appointments chairside at the end of an appointment. Chairside terminals also enable clinical staff to be the ones entering all treatment plans rather than the business staff. Clearly, because of its ability to relieve portions of the workflow for front desk people and the business staff, chairside terminals translate into lots of time saved for the front desk or business area. This allows them time to work on overdue accounts and overdue patients.

To Escort or Not to Escort

Some offices prefer that patients be escorted to the front desk. The less confusion up there, the better, particularly since clinical staff outnumber business staff by about three or four to one.

If the patients carry their own charts, the business staff is assured that both the charts and patients arrive back at the desk at the same time. A chronic complaint of the business staff is having patients at the desk without their charts. If this is a problem at your office, follow the Golden Rule of dynamic dentistry: The dental chair cannot go into an upright position until the paperwork is completed. Some offices have misgivings about patients carrying charts because they fear the patients will read them. In fact, they will, so here is another Golden Rule of dynamic dentistry: Never write anything in a chart you wouldn't want the patient to read.

We all love to press the chair button and bring the patients up. Tempting as it may be, don't rush things. Doctors, when you walk out of the treatment room, simply say to the patient, "Linda, I want you to relax for two or three minutes while Debbie finishes the paperwork (or the computer entries). Debbie's going to take over and tell you exactly what we've done today and what you can expect on your next visit."

One of the worst things that can happen at the front desk is when a patient pops out of a dental chair and comes right out front with no chart, no computer routing slip, and no other human being. The front desk person stands there and grins, filling time, "Hi, Mrs. Williams. How was your visit?" And so they chit-chat, until the front desk person says, "Excuse me," and runs into the back to play a game I call "Chase the Chart."

In reappointing, the scheduling coordinator at the front desk should ask, "Are mornings or afternoons better for you?" If the question is phrased, "When would you like to come in?" the patient might take ten minutes to decide. If the patient responds that mornings are best, the scheduling coordinator should offer a choice of two morning appointments that need to be filled by saying, "The doctor can see you Wednesday the 4th at 10:30 or Thursday the 5th at 11:00." This is how scheduling coordinators control their schedule rather than permit the schedule to control the practice! It also eliminates prime time appointments being filled weeks in advance with openings at non-prime time tomorrow and the next day.

When you present the fee, stand up and look directly at the patient and say, "Marsha, your fee for today is 225. Will that be cash, check, or bank card?" Do not ask, "Would you like to pay any of that today?" Marsha may very well say NO. Do not even include phrases like "Would you like" or "How would you like" in presenting fees.

The business staff member will have better results when dealing with patients who have no insurance if she presents fees in positive terms such as "Your fee today is eighty-five. Will that be cash, check, or bank card?" If three "Yes" answers are offered, one will usually result. Never say "dollars" as it is a negative, turn-off word. The business staff member should say, "Your fee today is three twenty-five" not "three hundred twenty-five dollars." And never say "hundred"—which can also be a turn off.

All instructions for posting and reappointment should be clearly written on the computer care slip by the chairside person. This saves time for the business staff when patients arrive at the desk. Since there are usually three or four clinical staff for every business staff, the more front desk time that can be saved, the better. This may seem like a duplication of duties chairside, but it only takes about forty seconds of the assistant's or hygienist's time. The information is fresh in their minds after charting and saves several minutes' research per patient at the front desk. For paperless practices, time in stopping at the business area is shortened or eliminated with "Quick Pay" chairside by credit card.

Phase Eight: Patient Exit

The last phase of patient communication, the exit, is extremely important; don't be tempted to think of this phase as a mere dismissal. The way a patient is handled when they're exiting is the patient's last impression of the office. The business staff member should tell the patient good-bye with words like, "Ms. Jones, it was nice seeing you today. We look forward to your visit next Thursday the 16th at 10:00."

New patients are the lifeblood of your practice, and this phase of communication is the perfect time to double new patient referrals by inviting family, friends, and co-workers of the patient to use the practice. The dynamic dentistry principle is simple: Invite, invite, invite!

If an insurance patient has good dental coverage, the financial coordinator may say, "Mr. Brown, I don't know if you are aware of it, but your dental plan is one of the best we see in this office. If your co-workers don't have a personal dentist, we'd be pleased to see them." Several studies have shown that thirty to forty percent of employees with employee benefit plans do not see dentists on a regular basis. Some of them need only to be invited. While many practices each year become insurance-free, that is, they no longer accept assignment of insurance benefits as payment for patient services, those practices that still accept insurance can increase patient flow with this type of invitation.

If the office has been seeing Mrs. Johnson and her children and she speaks of her husband, the scheduling coordinator may say, "Mrs. Johnson, we haven't had the pleasure of meeting Mr. Johnson. If he isn't seeing another dentist, we'd love to meet him." It should become the goal of each staff member to invite patients into the practice. Inviting is not soliciting or selling; it's merely being conscientious and concerned.

The Bottom-Line Impact of Delegation

Dentists spend an average of ten minutes per patient talking dentistry, which includes social interaction and all the pre- and post-treatment explanations.

In most practices, the staff spends about twenty-five percent of its time with patients talking about dentistry and the balance in social conversation. These percentages must be reversed: staff should spend seventy-five percent of their time with patients talking about dentistry and the balance in social conversation. The means for enabling this to happen is delegation. The dentist needs to shift responsibility for much of the pre- and post-treatment explanation to staff.

Why? Some simple math tells the story most effectively:

Calculate the average number of patients—including hygiene—seen in your office each day. Multiply the daily total by the number of days in which the practice sees patients. Divide by the number of dentists in the practice, for example:

> 60 patients X 16 days = 960 per month/2 dentists = 480 patients per month each X 7 minutes = 3,360 minutes/60 = 56 hours/16 per month = 3.5 hours per day per doctor

If the dentist delegates seventy percent of patient education to the staff, this saves seven of the ten minutes the dentist spends on average with each patient.

The answer usually ranges from two to four hours or more. This means that the average dentist spends from two to four hours each day talking to patients...not treating them, that is, generating revenue, but simply providing pre-treatment explanations and post-treatment reassurances, communication that can be delegated. Out of all the office staff, the dentist's time is the most expensive, which means having him or her conduct the majority of this non-revenue generating conversation is about as costly as time gets in a dental practice.

Once the dentist and the staff harmonize this process, that is to say, once they develop a strategy of having the staff take over the pre-treatment explanation and the post-treatment reassurances—and train the staff to do it with confidence and competence (see Clinical Cue Cards, below)—productivity, and with it profitability, soars.

Some more math: Once this time (seven minutes per patient multiplied by the average daily number of patients divided by sixty) is freed up, calculate the savings by multiplying this figure by the doctor's hourly production of $300 to $600 per hour. You will see, as our clients have seen, that your practice can increase from $800 to $1,800 a day!

Using $800 a day for illustration, this amounts to $160,000 a year on a 200-day year. On an $1,800 per day increase, this is $360,000.

While I never want to take away the joy of doctor to patient communication, you can see that talking and patient education is expensive if the dentist is doing all the talking.

No one in the office can do clinical restorative dentistry except the doctor. This is why every minute counts in time management and scheduling. When a dentist says, "But communicating with my patients is the most enjoyable part of practicing," I say, "Fine doctor, as long as you don't mind losing about $160,000 per year doing it!" A dentist might say, "But Linda, my patients want ME to do everything for them," or "My patients want to hear it from ME, not my staff." My response is, "In due respect, Doctor, as long as you think that way, they will." Delegation and effective time management are the reasons a solo practice can now produce six figures per month in a four-day week versus the stagnant $50,000 per month practice that works longer hours, more days, and has much more stress, mostly related to overhead!

And honestly, when I ask any doctor whether after seeing that figure he or she has any hesitation delegating pre-treatment explanation and post-treatment reassurances to staff, I'm likely to hear something like, "For $160,000 a year, I think I can let go of it."

Clinical Cue Cards

Doctors should create what I call clinical cue cards for training the team to have pre- and post-treatment conversations with patients. Be sure, by the way, that everyone uses these clinical cue cards: from the newest hire to the employee with the longest service. Each staff member should memorize the cards as quickly as possible, and then they should be saved for the next new hire.

One set is the pre-treatment explanation cards. On these cards, doctors put a procedure: porcelain inlays, composite restoration, three-unit bridge, etc., along with precisely what needs to be said to the patient prior to the presentation of each of these procedures, including especially the value or the benefits of the procedure for the patient.

We can talk until we're blue in the face about the importance of replacing a missing tooth, but until you outline the short- and long-term importance of investing in a three-unit bridge or an implant to replace a missing tooth, I guarantee they will say, "Well, that tooth has been out a long time and I've never missed it, so why bother?"

The second set of cards are post-treatment reassurance cards. These include what the dentist would say after explaining, "Linda, it was great seeing you today. I look forward to your next visit. I'm going to turn you over to Wendy. Wendy is my chairside assistant, and she will be explaining exactly what we've done today, and she'll answer any questions you may have."

As with the pre-treatment explanation cards, put a procedure at the top of each card and precisely what needs to be said to the patient at the end of each of these procedures, especially what the patient should expect in terms of soreness, sensitivity, and the like.

Remember that clinical cue cards are for everyone, not just the clinical staff, but the business staff as well. Business staff must have sets of clinical cue cards since they often receive clinical questions from patients. Their knowledge level is significant in the patient's mind.

The primary purpose of these clinical cue cards is to provide the means to enable everyone on the team to "sing from the same sheet of music" and ensure high standards and consistency in the practice's patient education efforts and replies to patient questions. In essence, the doctor's words come from the lips of every staff member.

In addition to producing significant savings to the practice each year, delegating pre- and post-treatment communication to the staff is important because it provides a kind of third party objective viewpoint and because it shows that the doctor trusts the team. This comes across to patients loud and clear and the result is that their trust and confidence increases too.

One endontic client put it best when she said, "The most exciting part is that you allowed me to get out of the treatment room very quickly. We've been able to trim ten minutes off every procedure, and I've added another molar endodonic procedure in the morning, and one in the afternoon. My production's up $1,400 a day because I'm not doing all the talking. More important than the money is the fact that my two assistants are on fire for dentistry. They were good assistants, but now they're exceptionally good assistants, because now they feel personally involved in the communication."

Special Situations

Special situations require expert handling and communication skills.

The Difficult Patient

The adage, "Two percent of patients cause ninety-eight percent of the stress" is often true. Here's the key, however: tempting as it may be, do your best not to dwell on the two percent. The challenges and difficulties they present will drain a disproportionate amount of your time and attention. You'll have less time and energy to focus on the ninety-eight percent who need and deserve your help.

Bear in mind that the majority of "two-percenters" don't intend to create stress; they simply do. They have extra demands and special needs. Perhaps they lack social skills. Do your best to look beyond these characteristics and perform your job to the best of your ability.

The Angry Patient

Occasionally a patient may become angry over a statement, a treatment misunderstanding, or the way the dentist or an employee behaved. Most angry situations can be resolved with empathy, consideration, and kindness. Teaching to "mood match" helps. If the patient speaks very fast, your deliberate slowing down in response will often slow down their speech. Breathing deeper and more slowly may in fact calm the patient. Using phrases such as, "I can understand how you feel," and "Please go over that again so that I may more clearly understand your viewpoint," sends a positive message that the patient's problem is now yours, and that you're concerned and interested in hearing the particulars.

Saying, "I'm sorry; that's the policy," or "You owe it and you must be responsible for it" only angers the patient more. This tone of voice says, "It's your problem. Now deal with it!"

The old strategy of "killing them with kindness" is more effective than a tart response that tends to escalate the anger even more. The dentist must demonstrate the particular brand of "kindness" in order for the staff to know this is the way these patients are to be handled. Statistics clearly state that sixty-seven percent of patient loss in dental practices is caused by rude, overbearing, uncaring employees—more than two-thirds! For this reason, the dentist should never ignore or defend an employee's rudeness.

All this notwithstanding, no member of the staff should accept verbal abuse from anyone. If the patient is having a bad day and wants the office to have one too, the dentist should step up to the plate and nicely yet firmly stand behind the staff one-hundred percent with phrases such as, "Mr. Jones, I'm sorry you aren't happy with our financial policy. Susan was just doing the job that we have hired her to do. In fact, the majority of our patients appreciate and respect the work Susan does for our practice. In future visits I hope you can do the same."

Allow the staff to know that in rare cases when they are confronted with an angry patient, the dentist will come to their rescue if their own attempts to cool the situation down are not effective. This is good management and it's also essential for making it clear to patients that while you sympathize with their frustration or disappointment, the practice has guidelines and procedures that will be followed even if a particular patient doesn't like them.

There's a major difference between standing behind the staff if they have handled the patients with dignity and respect while enforcing the guidelines in a very friendly way and simply allowing rude and discourteous behavior to patients.

The Patient Who Refuses to Pay

Having clear written financial guidelines is the first step in alleviating patient non-compliance when it comes to paying for services rendered. Many practices do not have written guidelines so the staff in these practices only guess at how to present and collect fees. In still other practices, the financial coordinator has had little if any training in financial verbal skills for discussing the fees or knowing positive fee rebuttals when patients refuse to pay at the time of service or by an agreed upon date.

Another essential step in collections is conveying a positive attitude regarding patient benefit plans. While the staff should be happy if the patient has an insurance plan that will provide partial reimbursement, knowing that patients are ultimately responsible for all fees related to their treatment enables the staff and dentist to stop making patients codependent on their insurance. If your office hears phrases such as "I only want to do what my insurance covers," or "Will this be covered by my insurance?" on a regular basis, chances are the office is routinely saying, "I'll have Susan check with your insurance to see what they will cover." (See Chapter 7 on pages 140-142 for more collection of fee information.)

The Frightened Patient

A patient may call the office and explain, "I just really don't like going to the dentist; it's taken me three years to make this call" or "I'm scared to death of dentists; my last experience was terrible." Make a practice of acknowledging these expressions of fear and low trust coming from a patient. They are very real and require special handling.

Never try to talk frightened patients out of fear as it only heightens it. Remember that kindness, concern, and even some empathy are more effective with a frightened patient than comments like, "You've got nothing to worry about as you'll be fine" and "Oh, Mr. Jones, there's nothing to a root canal, in fact, it's no worse than a filling." These sorts of comments do nothing to help fearful patients, but instead make them feel as if their fears are unwarranted. To the frightened patient, fear is real and larger than life. In addition, in reality neither the patient nor the staff really knows that everything will be fine until the treatment is done, making these empty promises that can undermine the patient's trust.

Express sympathy by saying, "We have a word that describes how you feel, Mr. Jones. That word is normal." Patients begin to relax when they feel they are understood; they feel safer and more secure. You might also want to try, "Mr. Jones, you've called the right office. We specialize in patients who have had less than ideal dental experiences in the past. In fact, one of our greatest compliments is having an apprehensive patient refer all their friends and relatives."

Mark or highlight the patient's name on the schedule and on his chart in a way that will enable everyone on the staff to know the patient is likely to need some extra time and attention. For instance, use the notation "TLC" by the name (tender loving care) so that everyone will know the patient needs to feel especially welcome and reassured.

When this notation is used on the scheduler before the patient comes in, the computer generates the notation on the daily work list the day of the appointment and thereby alerts the entire staff to the fearful patient who needs extra TLC. If you have a morning huddle at the start of each day, identify and briefly discuss these patients during the meeting and discuss ways to provide the type of TLC and support they may need.

The Late Patient

We get treated in life the way we teach people to treat us. As it is with individuals, so it is with dental practices. What on earth am I talking about? Simply this: when you respect the schedule, patients will too. I have found in office after office that when the practice consistently runs behind schedule, late patients and cancellations are prevalent. Patients cannot be expected to be on time if they have been kept waiting to see the dentist or hygienist in the past. In contrast, when appointments follow the schedule closely, patients arrive promptly and cancellations are minimal. Patients follow the cues of the office—for better or worse.

Any dental office that expects its patients to be on time for their appointments must have policies that demonstrate to the patient that their time is also respected and considered valuable. Like many of the challenging situations that arise in dental practices, the key to handling lateness on the part of patients is preparation. In the case of tardiness in particular, solid policies are essential.

Some examples:

Policy 1. If the doctor or hygienist is five minutes late, the person at the front desk must acknowledge the tardiness to the patient with an apology and an estimate of the remaining wait time. I've found that patients kept waiting are far less likely to be hostile if they're given a simple apology and an explanation of the situation.

Policy 2. If the doctor or hygienist is ten minutes late, he or she must go into the reception room and apologize in person to the waiting patient.

With these policies in force, I guarantee that the office will never be more than nine minutes behind schedule!

Specific policies should be in place for handling patients who arrive late for their appointments.

Some examples:

1. If a patient is habitually late, I recommend writing the time of the appointment ten minutes earlier on the appointment card than on the schedule. For example, write "10:50" on the card and enter "11:00" in the computer. If the patient arrives "on time" once or twice, since they've kept the office waiting many times in the past, it's okay to make them wait ten minutes or so in hopes that they develop better time habits. Offer to serve them coffee or juice as they wait. In fact most practices that serve beverages or have a self-serve adult beverage center like the first class airline lounges have patients coming in ten minutes early for this treat!

2. Have the following message printed on the patient brochure and appointment cards: "We value our patient's time and go out of our way to see them promptly. We appreciate the same promptness from our patients."

3. Develop an office policy that doctors and staff are comfortable with

for managing very tardy patients. I recommend rescheduling patients if they are late for more than half their appointment times. If a patient has a fifty minute appointment in the hygiene department and shows up thirty minutes late, the hygienist has three options: (1) elect to do half the prophy and reschedule the rest; (2) do a rush job in less than half the allotted time, running into the next patient's appointment time; (3) reschedule the patient for another time. Rescheduling is usually the best choice.

Don't be tempted to select options 1 or 2. Patients who receive half a prophy or a rushed job are likely to be angered by such treatment. They may say to the dentist, "Well, I certainly hope I don't get such a rush job on my next appointment." Rescheduling is the best choice. This is one of those "darned if you do and darned if you don't" situations. Knowing just what to say and how to say it to the late patient is a skill to be developed just like any other skill.

Unforeseen events and emergencies can disrupt the schedule of any dental office once in a while. But if the office runs behind and keeps patients waiting more than ten percent of the time in an eight hour day, this translates into forty-eight minutes of time. Over the course of 200 working days per year, this amounts to 160 hours of time.

You can easily monitor your on-time efficiency with the on-time monitor form. Copies can be downloaded from my website: wwwdentalmanagementU.com. After gathering this information, the team must meet to determine the causes and action steps that can be taken to alleviate the problem.

CHAPTER 3

Dynamic Staffing: Teams Work

Dynamic Dentistry is a book about high levels of success...about the strength and growth of a dental practice, and not just any practice—but yours. Of course, this kind of success doesn't happen by itself; it's the result of many factors working in concert. Of these many factors, inspired staffing and the teamwork it makes possible are among the most important.

Inspired?

Yes, inspired. Selecting, motivating, and managing a team of people demands nothing less than sharp insight into what makes people tick, who's well suited to perform specific tasks, both clinical and administrative, the types of people who work best together, and the quality of communication that forms the foundation of every aspect of people development and team building.

How do you develop this type of insight? You start with the realization that you don't find great teams of people, you create them. Experience plays a role, but so do certain tools, tips, and tactics that enable you to find and keep the sorts of professionals who become your practice's greatest asset.

The right people, working well not just as individual contributors but as a team—that's the formula. Read that sentence again: "The right people, working well not just as individual contributors but as a team…" The quality of teamwork a group is capable of is almost more important than an individual's ability to contribute on his or her own.

"Whoa there! That's a pretty big statement, Linda," you might say, and you'd be right. But the fact of the matter is, if people don't work well together by virtue of their natural temperament and the ways they respond to the environment in your office, key opportunities are lost and time and money are wasted since even the simplest tasks take longer to complete. I've seen dental practices make mistakes, communicate ineffectively, and order duplicate supplies because communication on the team was so poor. Anything and everything is harder to accomplish on a team whose players respond to the situations and circumstances that naturally arise in the course of running a dental practice in ways that pluck each other's last nerve.

The fact is that anyone can work together. Put six people in almost any setting and they will work together. But if those six people are not well chosen for both their skills and complementary behavioral styles, it will be impossible for them to work as a team. Ultimately, each person will simply be going through the motions of the work day, perhaps completing what's on the day's To-Do list, putting just enough energy into the job to get it done—and not one calorie more.

The office will function at the lowest level: just enough to get by. This low energy and negativity exacts a high price on any business, but it's all the more damaging in dentistry. A dental practice serves patients, and when a team isn't working in harmony, patients sense the tension and it heightens their anxiety. In most practices, there are few if any walls to hide behind; the reception desk is right out in front, visible and within earshot of patients. This means patients are in effect part of the office environment from the moment they enter the reception area. It's all out there—every bit of positive and negative energy—for every patient to see and experience from the time they walk in the door to the time they leave.

Dentistry is a people business, one of the caring professions. The dentist's, assistant's, and hygienist's clinical skills are essential, no question, but the quality of the patient's total experience is just as essential. It's human nature for patients to judge the quality of care by what they see and sense when they walk in the door, and to judge the unknown—the procedure they're about to undergo—by the total quality of the experience of being served by the practice.

The long-term prospects for such a poorly run practice would not be very bright, all because teamwork is impossible when people's behavioral styles don't mesh. After all my years of helping thousands of dental practices to improve everything from scheduling to collections, I've become convinced that poor or nonexistent teamwork is the root cause of most problems in an office.

Unless staff is carefully selected based on skills, experience, and behavioral style, all your efforts at teambuilding will be for naught, because both research and my own experience show that people whose behavioral styles are incompatible will never work together as a high performing team—ever. No matter how hard you try, no matter how many bonuses and incentives you provide to encourage teamwork, no matter how many team meetings you have, staff members' different behavioral styles will clash, conflicts will inevitably arise, and success will elude the practice year after year.

These are the reasons one of my favorite sayings is, "A team will outperform a group of individuals...every time."

The difference between a team and a group of individuals is easy to spot. In a group of individuals, each member:

- ✧ focuses on individual goals and individual glory
- ✧ has members who don't want to share the credit for achievements
- ✧ is focused on their own needs
- ✧ cannot see a common goal but instead just their own goal
- ✧ cannot focus long enough on making anyone else better because they're so focused on themselves
- ✧ may be threatened by the leader, and may therefore undermine the leader's success in big and small ways

✧ may confuse the patient by disagreeing with each other in front of him and bad-mouthing each other to patients

A team does the opposite in every respect. A team:

✧ learns from each other

✧ picks each other up

✧ sublimates ego for the good of the team

✧ sees and believes in a common goal

✧ anticipates and makes up for each other's weaknesses

✧ knows how to make everyone around them perform better

✧ supports the leader

✧ presents one unified, clear voice to the patient, keeping disagreements and squabbles behind closed doors

Why do teams consistently outperform groups of individuals? One word: synergy. The synergy principle states that "The whole is greater than the sum of the parts." When we apply this principle to teamwork, we see that through synergy, teams accomplish more and learn more in the process than a group of individuals. Teams have more creative ideas, experiences, and viewpoints to apply to any situation or tackle any problem, because one idea sparks another and another. Solutions grow; problems are easily solved through the collective brainpower of team members.

A dynamic dental practice works together synergistically, which means it operates at a higher level than just being in the same place at the same time doing related work. It functions synergistically…staff members work together freely, take responsibility, and–lest we forget–actually have fun.

The DiSC™ Profile

How do you find the right people for your practice and turn them into a high-performing team? The answer gets to the essence of leadership and management. The leader in you recruits and selects the right person. The manager in you establishes a positive work environment and builds a team of coworkers with complementary skills, experience, and behavioral styles to turn each person into a superior performer who increases the profitability and success of the practice as a whole.

So, let's start with finding the right people. The right people bring to the practice the right mix of skills and behavioral styles. Because they are objective and easily measured, skills are the easy part. You know the practice needs a talented patient coordinator, a superior hygienist, a talented financial coordinator, and exceptionally trained chairside assistants. You recruit candidates based on parameters for the number of years experience you want, clinical degrees, and other education requirements and the like, eliminating any candidates whose credentials fall short of your parameters.

Behavioral styles are both the tougher and, as I've suggested, the more important part. To find the people truly suited to your practice, you must determine how they will react to stimuli in your environment—including the dentist and other existing members of the staff—as well as how they will interact with patients.

There are any number of behavioral style assessment tools available to help you make this determination. Behavioral profiling is among them. I became an enthusiast of using behavioral profiles to help with hiring decisions back in 1982 when I was exposed to one such tool, the DiSC™ Profile, in a seminar I was attending. DiSC stands for Dominance, Image/Influence, Steadiness, and Conscientiousness, and the DiSC Profile is a highly accurate means of determining the ways in which an individual is likely to respond to people and situations in a work environment.

I completed my own DiSC Profile at the seminar and was astonished to see just how accurate it was. I've been even more astonished since at its accuracy and value in dental practice building. And unlike some other tools used to identify behavioral styles, the DiSC Profile is simple, highly accurate, and inexpensive. (For much more on the DiSC Profile, including ordering information for your office, visit www.dentalmanagementU.com to run your own workshop in your office.)

The DiSC Profile isn't something you pass or fail, and since results depend upon your environment, you can complete a profile six months or six years from now and it may very well be different. To complete the profile, you answer 10 to 28 questions from the perspective of how you'd respond to a number of situations in a work environment. Your responses provide information on how you solve problems, approach challenges, influence others, manage information, function within a certain structure, adapt to change, and in general meet the demands of your environment. The final output is a style designation that indicates your predominant style and strongest behavioral tendencies; you are either a D, I, S, or C. Each has a profile associated with it that outlines the individual's:

- ✧ Psychological need (that which satisfies the person within)
- ✧ Predominant strength (strengths that are apparent to others)
- ✧ Driving force (real passion)
- ✧ Greatest fear (hidden insecurities)
- ✧ Response to pressure (behavior when things go wrong)

The DiSC Profile has been validated in numerous studies, which means it's been proven to accurately predict the ways in which a person will respond to various situations and pressures in his environment. As a validated tool, the profile has high predictive value and can be used to match an applicant's style to the needs of the office.

High D

People whose predominant style is D are extroverted and task-oriented. Here is their profile:

Psychological Need:	To direct or dominate others
Predominant Strength:	High ego strength and task orientation
Driving Force	Personal challenges
Greatest Fear:	Being taken advantage of
Response to Pressure:	Impatience

If you are a high D, you have high ego strength. You like you. This is a positive quality because in my experience, if you don't like you, most other people won't either. High Ds are born leaders. They're goal-oriented, they want results, and they need variety in their work. High D's are easily bored by routine. They like to face new challenges on a regular basis. They have a basic fear of being taken advantage of and losing control. Their greatest weakness is that under pressure they may show a lack of concern for others' views or feelings.

A D will tell somebody something negative and feel absolutely no animosity toward them and then wonder why the person leaves the room sobbing. A D is direct and decisive and can make good decisions on very few facts. Some people call D's domineering. I call them leaders.

High I

People whose predominant style is I are extroverted and people-oriented. Here is their profile:

Psychological Need:	To interact with others
Predominant Strength:	Optimistic and people-oriented relaters
Driving Force	Social recognition
Greatest Fear:	Social rejection
Response to Pressure:	Disorganized

If you are a high I, you're extremely optimistic. You never see the glass as half empty; it's always three quarters full. An I loves to come up with great ideas and gets annoyed if you don't find their ideas to be spectacular. I's are highly people-oriented and for this reason, they tend to work exceptionally well in people-oriented businesses. They are motivated by social recognition such as awards and other forms of recognition for their contributions. It's easy to see why their greatest fear is that of not being liked.

You can tell if your children have high I tendencies; they always ask for two cookies or treats so they can give one to a friend. They are the most generous of all the behavioral styles; they'll give you the shirt off their backs in order to make you like them.

Under pressure, I's tend to become forgetful and disorganized. They may lose things or forget where they parked in the garage. This is one reason I's—if they want to be efficient—need to surround themselves with people who are highly organized.

I's are motivators and they keep the atmosphere at the office light and lively. But heaven help you if you put two I's in the same part of the office. You want to have one in the front and one in the back—and not too close together. If they're too close together, they'll spend most of their time patting each other on the back and having a good ol' sociable time every day, but rarely get anything done!

High S

People whose predominant style is S are introverted and people-oriented. Here is their profile:

Psychological Need:	To serve others
Predominant Strength:	Team player, loyal, and concrete results oriented
Driving Force	Traditional practices
Greatest Fear:	Loss of stability
Response to Pressure:	Possessiveness

High S's love consistent performance. They like to perform tasks the same way each time. Consistency appeals to them in policies, methods of completing tasks, standards, and measures...nearly every aspect of what they do. S's are also the most team-oriented of all the behavioral styles, which as I've said, is a wonderful quality, so important to have on staff.

S's are motivated to maintain the status quo. They like things to be organized and they like them to be right. The S's basic fears are loss of stability or security and change. They are the most change resistant people in the office.

Because S's are such wonderful people and it's hard to find anything wrong with them, the S profile person will become the head cheerleader in the face of change if they trust the person who's asking them to make the change and understand the reasons change is needed.

If your office is expanding or changing in any way and you have lots of

S's on staff, you're going to throw them too many curve balls and keep them stirred up a lot. Here's the guideline: Never spring a sudden decision on an S. For instance, if your financial or scheduling coordinator is an S and you turn to that person and say, "I just got back from this wonderful meeting, and we're going to have a new computer in here in two weeks," the S will just die. A far better approach is to say to the S, "You know, I'm thinking seriously about updating our computer systems, and we're going to do some research for the next ninety days. You'll be totally involved in the research, and you will actually help me select the system." The S will be fine with that because for S's, change in itself is not the problem...sudden change that takes place without their involvement is.

High S's basic fear is loss of security and stability. Under pressure, they can become over-willing to give advice, and so S's are your best counselors. If you need a shoulder to cry on, go to an S. They listen to everybody's problems.

High C

People whose predominant style is C are introverted and task-oriented. Here is their profile:

Psychological Need:	To comply with their own high standards
Predominant Strength:	Accuracy and highly intuitive
Driving Force	Correct or proper way
Greatest Fear:	Criticism of their work
Response to Pressure:	Overly critical

The high C is analytical and has a high attention to detail. I've said many times in my seminars that if you want something done right, hire a C. They're very task-oriented and they love to create and follow checklists. They're also motivated by correctness and quality. Their basic fear is criticism of their work. The reason that is a basic fear for them is that they try so hard to do it right every single time.

If you can get the high C's on the team to moderate their attention to detail a bit and get the rest of the staff to sharpen their attention to detail, the team can work in harmony. But if your high C's expectations are left unchecked and the balance of the team's expectations are not as strong, there will definitely be problems in the form of tension and disagreement.

You might want to have a Popsicle stick with the words "chill out" on it that you jokingly hold over the heads of your high C's—out of the view of patients of course!—just to keep the environment light when these folks become too detail-oriented and perfectionistic.

Under pressure, high C's become even more perfectionistic and tend to be overly critical, of themselves and everyone around them. Consider the effects of this type of reaction to stress in a business like ours, filled with pressure almost every minute. You've got to be aware of your high C's and help them work within the pressure cooker of a dental practice effectively…for their own sakes, and for the sake of the practice as a whole. No one and nothing functions well when it's overly criticized, making this tendency seriously deleterious to the health and growth of a dental practice.

Once you go through the DiSC Profile process, you will become so accustomed to thinking in terms of the high D, I, S, and C profiles that even without profiling someone using the formal tool, you'll know very quickly what the person's predominant style is.

Getting into an elevator on a busy morning, the D walks up to the elevator and, even if the light is already on, punches it three more times. Slightly impatient. The I holds the door for everybody else, welcomes them on board, and chats with them all the way up or down. The S holds the door open and lets everyone else get on; if it fills up too quickly, he waits for the next one. The C jumps on first and stands in front of the control buttons, counts everybody that gets on, adds up their body weights, looks at the weight capacity number, and jumps off if the elevator is too full.

It's always amazing to me that without even profiling an audience, based on their response to my seminar I can tell you what their profile is. The I's and the S's are the warm and fuzzy people who say, "Loved your stories. I may have forgotten the point you were making, but I'll never forget your stories."

And I'll get a comment from a high D or high C such as, "Liked the program, but next time leave off the stories." They don't like all that soft stuff. Bottom line is that I can tell your behavioral style by how you like my behavioral and presentation style, and you'll find you develop the same quick perception and insight into the behavioral styles of the people in your professional and even your personal circles.

The DiSC Profile works! One female practitioner who had a first-class practice in a downtown exclusive neighborhood knew her business staff didn't truly share her vision nor were they performing their daily tasks adequately. She sought out and found what she needed—a DI office administrator with S and C tendencies—and the practice flourished within three months—a $28,000 per month increase in production!

The consultants were praised to the hilt for "fixing" this practice, but it was the strong leadership of the dentist who found and hired her practice's "missing link" that really turned the practice around on a dime.

Strategies for Working Effectively with Different Behavioral Styles

D = DOMINANCE

✧ Get to the point; be brief and specific.

✧ Avoid small talk, stick to business.

✧ Be prepared and well organized.

✧ Be confident; present logically and concisely.

✧ Ask specific questions.

✧ Provide choices and alternatives.

✧ Furnish facts concerning success probability, effectiveness, and longevity.

✧ Persuade and motivate by referring to results and objectives.

✧ After presentation, promptly and courteously depart.

I = INFLUENCING

✧ Get on their level; relate presentation to their lifestyle, work, and language.

✧ Allow time for socializing.

✧ Make presentation stimulating, friendly, and fast-moving.

✧ Don't overload them with extensive details; put them in writing.

✧ Strive for a commitment.

✧ Provide ideas for implementing treatment plan.

✧ Furnish testimonials; supply photographs.

✧ Offer incentives for immediate acceptance.

S = STEADINESS

✧ Start with personal commitment; break the ice.

✧ Show sincere interest; find areas of common involvement.

✧ Listen; be responsive.

✧ Present case softly, non-threateningly.

✧ Present in an informal but orderly manner.

✧ In an assuming manner, provide benefits of treatment.

✧ Do not rush through the presentation or rush into a commitment.

✧ Do not overwhelm—go slowly and allow time for patient to trust your judgment.

✧ Provide guarantee that their decision will minimize risks.

C = COMPLIANCE

✧ Prepare your case well ahead of time; be accurate.

✧ Stick to business; use a straightforward, direct, but low-keyed approach.

✧ Build credibility by listing pros and cons to any recommendation you make.

✧ Draw up a scheduled approach to implementing the treatment plan with step-by-step timetable.

✧ Use chairside communication and patient education props to provide solid, tangible, practical evidence.

My Profile

Completing the DiSC Profile is a revealing experience, so revealing in fact that it can sometimes make you uncomfortable. Once you complete it, you'll know more about yourself than your mother knows about you, including some things you may not like.

In fact, when I personally completed the DiSC Profile for the first time in 1982, I remember telling my husband about it. "I was in the most fascinating workshop today," I told him. "We completed something called the DiSC Profile that reveals our predominant behavioral style. It's about 98 percent accurate."

"How do you know it's only 98 percent accurate?" he asked.

"Well, there were two things on there that weren't true," I explained. "It said I was stubborn and hard-headed."

"Oh, well then it's one-hundred percent accurate!" he said.

Chances are, like me, you'll learn some things about yourself that you probably don't want to admit.

Until I was profiled for the first time in 1982, I was not aware of my strengths and weaknesses or how to tone down the strengths and work on the weaknesses as needed. As a chairside assistant, they called me "Chatty Cathy." I was one of those clinical team members who said, "There's not enough money in the world to pay me to work at the desk."

Learning that I was a high I with S tendencies helped me to finally understand why I loved the business side of dentistry so much. I got paid to TALK to patients all day! But I also realized that in order to get all my work done, I had to become more focused and less sociable. Without the DiSC profile, I'd have been frustrated and confused all these years.

The Effective Office

I use the DiSC Profile in making hiring decisions about candidates who apply to work at my company, and I strongly encourage you to do the same for your dental practice. The Profile helps you understand yourself and others, to recognize and therefore have the information you need to solve problems on your team once and for all, and to plan a staff of people with behavioral styles that work well together. And this can go beyond the daily grind of getting things done to see and capitalize on new opportunities like new technology, opportunities to expand the practice by hiring an additional hygienist or assistant, or even to add a new plant or change a piece of artwork in the reception area, for example.

In structuring the best possible team for your dental practice, bear in mind that people with similar behavioral styles tend to be compatible. In other words, if you and I have the same predominant behavioral style—we're both D's, I's, S's, or C's—we're likely to get along well and do great things together on the job.

On the other hand, mixing the different styles is likely to result in conflict in the office. Team members will disagree on the best approach to problem solving and have different responses to the daily stress of running a dental practice. They most likely will not get along well and the atmosphere and effectiveness of the office will not be optimal as a result.

The profile gives you the information you need to understand why we like to work with certain people and why we clash with others. Conflicts arise when we don't respect the differences—and of course that begins with understanding the differences. The DiSC behavioral profile will teach us that we will not respond to situations in the same way for very specific reasons. This doesn't mean that one of us is right and the other wrong but rather that our behavioral styles cause us to react differently to different stimuli.

If you decide to purchase DiSC Profiles for your office and it turns out that styles on the team are not compatible, don't go out and fire everyone! Try instead to first spend some time understanding the source of problems and then begin to create strategies and levels of awareness aimed at working together more effectively based on what you now know about each other. This means being more tolerant and forgiving.

Cultivate the three qualities that enable dissimilar teams to work together effectively:

- ✧ Mutual respect for one another, (No single member of the team is more important than another. Everyone has a crucial role to play in building success.)
- ✧ Mutual trust of one another, (Respect breeds trust. Once team members genuinely respect each other, they naturally trust each other's judgment and integrity.)
- ✧ A willingness to adapt, (Specifically, to another person's mood or habits. Anticipate their responses and reactions, and accept them…This is the essence of adaptability in a team environment.)

No Perfect Team

Understanding these behavioral profiles is essential to appreciating differences, heading them off at the pass, and learning to staff appropriately, and while there is no perfect team in a dental practice, the most efficient and effective offices are filled with people with a variety of styles that complement each other. Here are some general guidelines for building a high potential, high performing team using the results of the DiSC Profile:

- ✧ Because S is the most team-oriented of all the behavioral styles, it's wonderful if you have fifty percent high S's on your team.
- ✧ Ten to fifteen percent of your staff should be a high D or a high C because you need at least one leader to make decisions on change and a perfectionist to make sure the changes are correct.
- ✧ You should have at least twenty-five percent I's on your team because without the I's the office environment is very tense and you can cut the stress with a knife.

The Compatibility Chart

Below is the DiSC Profile Compatibility Chart, a summary of the styles and how they affect one another in social and work related situations.

DiSC Profile Compatibility Chart

	1	2	3	4	5	6	7	8
D-D				S	W			
D-I			S			W		
D-S	W					S		
D-C						W		S
I-I	S						W	
I-S	W				S			
I-C			W				W	
S-S	S		W					
S-C	S	W						
C-C	S		W					

Key: S= Social Interaction W=Work Tasks 1=Best Possible 8=Poorest Possible

As you review the chart, notice that, for example, two Ds are good together because they enjoy each other's determination, directness, and challenging personality. For these reasons, they like to be together socially. At work, however, the story's a bit different. On the job, two Ds are only a fair match because they clash; they both want to be in charge.

A D and an I are a better combination on the job. The I is the creative one; he or she comes up with ideas, and the I appreciates the D's ability to act on those ideas. Sounds like a good combination, and in general, it is. However, they can be a poor working team on the job because the D and the I have the same problem: they operate on the "Ready, fire, aim" principle. That is, they sometimes act impulsively. What would help? Some Cs and some Ss on the team.

The D and the S are a perfect work team. The D tells the S what to do and the S does it well. On a social level, a D and an S only tolerate each other; the D thinks the S is too slow and the S thinks the D is domineering. They probably won't be great friends, but on the job they're an unbeatable team.

A D and a C are potentially the least effective combination of profiles. The D thinks the C is too detail-oriented, and the C thinks the D is impetuous. The D says, "Let's go!" while the C says, "We need to do more research!"

Two I's together are the happiest of all on a social level because they enjoy dressing, talking, and entertaining. Let the C's and the S's get the work done.

An I and an S form the perfect work team because the I's generate the great ideas and the S's implement them. On a social level, the S's tolerate the Is. They may sometimes think, "NOT another idea! We haven't finished the other two we're working on."

I and C together form a solid work team. The C keeps the I on-task, making sure the I is doing the job well, not being too creative, but focusing on the practical too.

S and S together are an excellent work team, though they are both somewhat resistant to change.

S and C together are absolutely dynamite on the job. The C's make sure the S's are not only task-oriented, but they do the work correctly.

C and C together are also an excellent work team: two perfectionists who know that they are the only two perfect people in the office.

Use It with Patients

The DiSC Profile is a powerful tool for selling dentistry and building patient relationships. If the dentist has one and only one way to present a treatment plan, fifty percent or more of patients are being lost. Fifty percent or more! This is because to sell effectively, you must tailor your case presentation to the patient's behavioral style: a D, I, S, or C.

In general, D's will want you to be direct, giving just the facts. S's and C's will need to know more specifics and the long-term benefit to the buyer. I's will be your best cosmetic cases because they're driven by image and influence. They'll need the dentist to supply information about their treatment plans by saying how attractive the end results will be. S's will need to have high trust in you before you present the plan. Never tell them they need a $7,000 treatment plan on the first, second, or third visit. A C will ask a lot of very technical questions. They'll need you to outline each detail of the treatment and provide before and after pictures how they will look post treatment.

Note: LLM&A has "Getting to Know You" cards that you can order on our website at www.dentalmanagementU.com to determine the patient's style by asking general dental related questions.

If you want to increase your closing ratio on treatment plans, start reading your patients and presenting treatment plans according to what they need to hear…not what you want to say. For example, let's say a treatment plan consists of four porcelain inlays on posterior teeth and eight veneers on the maxillary anteriors.

To present this plan to a D you'd say:

> *"Mr. Jones, I'll cut through the chase of the types of porcelains and labs we use, just to say that by removing the old restorations that have outlived their usefulness and replacing them with inlays, plus placing eight veneers on your anterior teeth, the results you desire will be there. I normally can't see a half day case for at least two weeks but you're in luck. I just had a change in my schedule for Thursday morning. See Mary up front. She'll go over the financial options and get you scheduled."*

Remember, with the D's, get to the point and leave the room in a busy practice to get the patients back quickly. These behavioral styles "cool off" and get busy and antsy if they're delayed in any way.

To present this plan to an I, you'd say:

> *"Mrs. Bailey, I know how important a healthy and attractive smile is to you. Besides restoring your teeth, the porcelain inlays and veneers will give you a smile you'll be proud to show off. You not only need a healthy and attractive smile, you deserve to do this for yourself."*

With the I's, don't forget to mention esthetics and the word deserve. These are the most generous of all behavioral styles, so taking care of themselves will take place when they feel it is deserved.

To present this plan to an S, you'd say:

"Mrs. Taylor, my main concern is the deterioration of those old restorations on the posterior teeth back there. Let's take the treatment plan one step at a time, explaining each step along the way and its benefit (short and long-term) to you. After we get through with Phase I of the plan, you and I will discuss your options for restoring your front teeth."

S's are the fifty percent of your patient base who go somewhere else for a second opinion if the trust level isn't there. Because they were told too much too soon, they walked. Let them know there's more, but it does not have to be presented all at once. Phased dentistry is a must with the S's.

To present this plan to a C, you'd say:

> *"Mr. Jordan, being the engineer that you are, you will appreciate the function that will be restored to your mouth when the old restorations are removed and the porcelain inlays are placed. We are very much into occlusion as well as esthetics in our practice. The veneers on your anterior teeth in the front are state of the art. After your impressions are sent to the best lab in Texas, your custom designed veneers will be fabricated to the exact model replica of your teeth. Mid-lines and centric relationships will be established, recorded, and transferred to the laboratory for the perfect end results."*

C's want four years (or more) of dental school in a five-minute discussion. They want to know the minute details of the procedure and the anticipated end results. They ask many questions and are the exact opposite of the D, who wants to know as little as possible. Just get it done!

Building Your Staff: Attracting Job Candidates

Now that you know how to determine the skill levels and behavioral styles of the people who will work well within your practice, you must go out and find them. The key to hiring employees who will become part of a dynamic, high-performing team is to have a good number of applicants to choose from.

An ad in the Help Wanted section of the local newspaper is one way to attract people. To attract dynamic potential staff members, your employment ads should contain phrases like: "Are you caring and enthusiastic?

Do you enjoy a challenge in the health care profession? Are you dependable and goal-oriented?" These phrases tend to attract job applicants who develop into great team members.

An advertisement listing the office telephone number has pros and cons. The pros include being able to screen the calls to determine the applicant's ability to talk comfortably on the phone and only schedule interviews with qualified applicants. The cons are that many unqualified applicants may call about the job and incoming applicant calls may interrupt normal tasks.

A "blind" ad—one that does not provide the practice's address or phone number—asks applicants to fax or e-mail their resumes and a cover letter. Career-minded applicants have solid resumes and know how to compose a good cover letter. Dental staff members must have initiative. Putting together a resume and composing a good cover letter are clear indications of this trait. The main downside of a blind ad is the risk of having one or more of your own staff apply for the position!

Read the following sample ads:

1.

> WANTED: Dental Assistant (part time). Are you an enthusiastic, experienced dental assistant with a caring manner? Are you dependable and organized? If so, please send resume to Box 523, c/o this paper.

2.

> WANTED: Dental Business Assistant (full time). Do you have excellent communication skills over the telephone and in person? Are you enthusiastic, caring, and dependable. If you have experience with appointment scheduling, insurance, and accounting, and you like working in an office that appreciates staff, please e-mail your resume to _________.

3.

> WANTED: Dental Hygienist (four days per week). If you are enthusiastic, caring, and dependable and you enjoy a challenge in a patient-centered practice, please call 481-2276 between 10:00 a.m. and noon only.

4.

> WANTED: Dental Assistant. Seeking an exceptional team person. We focus on warmth, caring, and expert communication. Emphasis on personal development through continuing education, participation with other team members, and high achievement. Applicant should be career-minded, personally stable, and health-centered in lifestyle. Call 497-8611.

Advertisement 1 is an example of a brief ad that deliberately leaves out office hours and location. If you list evening and Saturday hours, for instance, you may reduce the number of applicants by as much as seventy-five percent. Again, your goal is to attract as many qualified applicants as possible. Sometimes, people like the job so much that the hours and location become irrelevant. In fact, some of the greatest success stories in hiring have been with staff members who traveled twenty-five to thirty miles to a particular job. Hours and distances are minor factors if the match is right.

Advertisement 2 may seem long, but I feel business assistants must have the most detailed ad. They not only should be good in business skills but in human skills as well. Too many offices concentrate on business skills—perhaps a high D—only to learn subsequently that their brand new Patient Coordinator is not a "people person." Others put a "charming hostess" up front—perhaps a high I—who within weeks is overwhelmed by the responsibilities of trying to please the doctor, staff, and patients. Spending a few extra dollars on an ad and then screening carefully will save you time, money, and stress.

Advertisement 3 is an example of a short positive ad that's also a marketing device. Here's how this works: when people move to new communities, they often read the Help Wanted section. Perhaps as they're looking for a position in their own field, they see an ad for a dental office that's "patient-centered" and decide to investigate for themselves. For this reason, this type of ad should include the office telephone number. To keep phone interruptions to a minimum, list the doctor's private number and have someone come in from 10:00 to noon to take the calls and screen the applicants. This keeps the calls from interrupting activities at the front desk (and if they call at any other time, that's an indication that they can't follow directions).

Advertisement 4 is positive and directed at a special, high achievement person. The money invested in the length of the ad saves many dollars' worth of time sifting through unqualified applicants.

Important!
I'm often asked whether the DiSC Profile is a legally approved, nondiscriminatory tool for making hiring decisions. The answer is yes, as long as it's used in conjunction with other hiring information such as the results of an applicant's personal interviews and a resume review. An applicant's DiSC Profile can't be used as the sole basis for making a hiring decision, nor can the profile be the reason a final hiring decision was made. In short, all an applicant's qualifications must be considered in making the final decision about whether to hire this person...which is just plain good business sense anyway!

Other Sources of Prospects

In addition to newspaper ads, consider these additional sources of auxiliary personnel:

Local Dental Auxiliary and Hygiene Associations

Within these groups there's sometimes an employment chairperson or networking contact. These individuals keep telephone numbers of staff seeking employment and a log of offices needing staff. This "matchmaker" is simply a contact person who provides services for which no fee is normally charged.

Dental Sales Representatives

This "through-the-grapevine" contact has proven beneficial because sales representatives sometimes know who is available, or will be available, before this information is public knowledge. For instance, a staff person may confide in a sales representative that she is contemplating a move. Subsequently, an office person three blocks away may say to the sales rep, "We're losing our number one assistant; be on the lookout for us" and bingo! Use these contacts to help you find candidates without having to spend time and money on employment ads.

Technical Schools

These are excellent sources of prospective employees. Notify the schools that the office is interested in hiring a recent or upcoming graduate. The alumni of these schools often place their names on the "available" lists when they are between positions, even after graduating.

Employment Agencies

Agencies that specialize in dental placements are often helpful, even though a fee is involved. If their pool of temporary and permanent placements is strong, the chances are good for finding a qualified staff member.

Beware of agencies that have a pool of untrained, low-qualified, unskilled workers. These types of agencies often charge high fees. Read the contract closely, ask questions, and check the agency's track record by asking for the telephone numbers of three offices that have used their services. If the agency says their policy is not to divulge client's names, keep looking. All reputable firms have happy clients willing to say, "You may use our name as a satisfied client."

Important!
Never take employees away from other dental practices. Actively seeking out and stealing another office's staff members with promises of higher pay or better benefits is unethical and will reflect poorly on the practice. I've actually overheard staff members asking, "If they would steal another office's staff, what else might they do that's unfair?"

However, if a staff member in office A is a friend of the hygienist in office B, the office A person is free to say, "Our hygienist is leaving in a month. Do you have any friends who may be interested in working here?" And if the office B hygienist then expresses personal interest in working in office A, it's completely ethical for her to be interviewed for the position.

In times of staff shortages, recruitment bonuses, including sign-on dollars or a week-long trip to Hawaii for two at the end of the first year, are not uncommon offerings from employers trying to lure good people from other offices.

I absolutely don't feel this is in anyone's best interest and it usually backfires in the loss of other good staff who were not given the same option when they were hired. Plus, it gives the new employee an attitude of "queen bee status" before their first day on the job.

Special Note on Inexperienced Applicants

An applicant's lack of experience shouldn't always be viewed as a negative. Some doctors say they'd rather create new habits than break old ones. In my mind, attitude should be considered first. If the applicant has a great attitude, he or she can learn to perform any job in the office.

Waitresses, for example, are a potential source of dental office personnel. Notice them when you are dining in nice restaurants. A waitress who cares about customers, smiles freely, and moves quickly and with dexterity may be receptive to a career in dentistry rather than a job. Many would gladly exchange weekend and evening hours on their feet in a restaurant for a career in a nice health care office. Many dentists report that some of their best employees have come from this tip.

Interviewing

Set an interview appointment for all qualified applicants. Allow your present staff to have some input in the hiring process. If a business staff person is being hired, have another business staff member take the top three applicants to lunch individually. If this isn't possible, have a present staff member participate in the preliminary interview. I have found that hard-working, industrious staff members will encourage only winners to join the team.

If you're looking to hire a hygienist or chairside assistant, allow a member of the clinical staff to participate in the selection process. When present staff participate in selecting a new employee, they tend to go out of their way to make a new person fit into the practice.

Interviews are time-consuming, but when they're done right, the rewards are well worth it.

Here are some helpful interview questions to use as guidelines as general interview questions. Ask conversation inspiring, open-ended questions:

1. Please describe your present responsibilities and duties.
2. How do you spend an average day?

3. How have you changed the content of your job from when you assumed it to now?
4. Discuss some of the problems you've encountered on the job.
5. What do you consider your chief accomplishment in your present job?

To determine qualifications the applicant has in addition to work experience, ask:

1. How do you view the job for which you are applying?
2. What in your background particularly qualifies you to do the job?
3. If you were to obtain this job, in what areas could you contribute immediately?
4. In what ways have your education and training prepared you for the job?

To probe for weaknesses:

1. What disappointments did you have in your previous job?
2. In what areas did you need help or guidance from your supervisor?
3. For what things has your supervisor praised you? Criticized you?
4. Of all the aspects of your last job, what did you like most? Least?

Questions designed to uncover the following specific qualities:

Motivation:

1. Why did you select this type of career?
2. What is it you seek in a job?
3. What is your long-term career objective?
4. What kind of position would you like to hold in five years? Ten?
5. What do you want in your next job that you are not getting now?

Stability:

1. What are your reasons for leaving your present job? Previous jobs?
2. Why are you seeking a job now?
3. What were your original career goals?

4. Have they changed?
5. What has been your greatest disappointment in terms of your career thus far?
6. How did it change your thinking?

Resourcefulness:

1. How did you change the scope of your previous job?
2. What were some of the difficult problems encountered on the job?
3. How did you solve them?
4. What do you know about our practice?
5. What do you know about the position you seek?
6. What are the three most important assets you bring to this office.
7. To whom did you go for counsel when you couldn't handle a job problem?
8. What kind of problems did you bring to this person?

Ability to Work Under Direction or with Others:

1. Describe your doctor's supervisory methods. Evaluate them.
2. For what things have you been complimented? Criticized?
3. On what committees have you served?
4. What did you contribute to each committee's work?
5. In your previous jobs, how much of your work was done on your own?
6. As part of a team?
7. What qualities do you seek in a boss?
8. What should your boss know about you to supervise you effectively?
9. What should your team members know about you to work with you effectively?

For Office Administrators:

1. Describe how you manage others.

2. How did you persuade the doctor to accept your new ideas?
3. Describe your technique of getting a job done.
4. What do you feel are the three key attributes of a successful practice administrator?

Specific job-related interview questions:

1. How did you approach some of the problems on your previous job?
2. What were the results?
3. In your previous job, what percentage of your time was spent on (name of duty)?
4. What experience do you have with (name a specific duty or responsibility)?
5. What were some of the significant achievements of your work group as a result of your efforts?
6. What aspects of this position will be new to you?
7. Which ones will require additional training, either on the job or technical, before you feel you can achieve proficiency?
8. Describe your strengths. Describe areas that need improvement, if any.

Remember, your interview questions should:

✧ assess only the knowledge, skills, abilities, and other work charactertics needed for entry-level performance or to learn the job, not those to be learned in training

✧ mirror the content of the job and fall into four basic categories: hypothetical, job knowledge, job simulation, or job sample, and work over requirements

✧ assess requirements in proportion to their relative importance to adequate job performance

✧ be precise, complete, and unambiguous to avoid the need for clarification that would disrupt standardization and introduce potential bias.

Employment Law

Familiarize yourself with state and federal laws and regulations that govern the hiring process. You should know that federal law prevails unless state laws give more rights to the employee. Contact your state and local government offices for copies of the statutes and regulations governing business practices, including the:

Civil Rights Act
Equal Pay Act
Age Discrimination Act
National Labor Relations Act
Freedom of Information Act
Pregnancy Discrimination Act
Uniform Guidelines
Sexual Harassment Guidelines

My friend and colleague Bent Ericksen of Bent Ericksen and Associates in California is a tremendous resource on hiring and dismissing employees, creating and maintaining employee files and manuals, and much more. See our website for his office policy manual and other useful products at www.dentalmanagementU.com.

Making the Offer

When you're ready to make the job offer, make it in writing. The letter should state the salary, hours, position, title, main job descriptions, date of hire, and benefits and should spell out any probationary period. Send two copies of the letter and ask the applicant to sign and return one copy for the office's files. If it is not feasible to send an offer letter, have the applicant sign the job description portion of the application as part of the hiring process. This helps prevent future misunderstandings about job responsibilities.

I recommend a ninety-day trial period for every new employee. This introductory period allows the office and the employee adequate time to determine if the applicant is suited for the job. During this ninety-day probationary period, the employee is ineligible for benefits. At the end of the trial period, the employee should receive an evaluation. If the evaluation is favorable, the employee is placed on regular status and furnished with a list of benefits.

You Must Staff Adequately

It's impossible to overstate the importance of adequate staffing. Too often, I've seen a patient leave a practice simply because the dental assistant has to be in two places at the same time, and the patient feels abandoned while the assistant is attending to another patient. Proper utilization of staff is not possible if one dental assistant has to run back and forth between treatment rooms.

You may be concerned about the expense of additional staff members, but view them as an investment.

The formula for adequate staffing varies by geography and type of practice. Some consultants will tell you not to staff by production, but by the number of people who check in and check out. I disagree with that because one patient may take thirty seconds to check out while one may take ten minutes. A far better measure of staffing needs is the type of dental practice. If you're a pediatric practice, the number of staff would be higher because you have to see a lot more little people to do the same volume production. If you're a periodontist, orthodontist, or endodontist, the number of staff would probably be lower. If you're in New York City versus Birmingham, I might suggest going by fees in your area. Fees are typically double in Manhattan what they are in many southern or midwestern states.

Clearly, staffing needs vary by the type of fees you're charging and the type of practice you run. If you see one $10,000 case for four hours in the morning, you certainly don't need as many support staff as a practice that sees twelve shorter appointments in the same time frame. As a general guideline, though, a practice needs one business staff person for each $40,000 to $50,000 a month in revenue. Here's an example of how to apply this information: if you have more than a $40,000 practice and you've got one person out front, to bring the practice up to the next revenue tier of $60,000 to $80,000, you must add one person. One person will be your scheduling and public relations coordinator while the other will be the practice's financial and insurance coordinator. Each of these positions require a minimum of eight hours per day to increase the revenue stream and serve patients completely.

"Frontdesklessness"
Some consultants and some dentists advocate "frontdesklessness," meaning exactly what it sounds like: all clinical staff are dually trained to check patients in and out. While this seems, in theory, workable, and it is in a small percentage of offices, it's also a hazard, and I know of a number of offices that have tried it without success.

Phones are often answered electronically, the patient coordinator greets the patients by remote camera, goes to the front area and brings the patient to the treatment room, stays with them throughout the treatment phase, and escorts them back to the front for check out. Who, then, is available to tear down the treatment room and sterilize it for the next patient? Who is doing the lab work and instruments from the last procedure, and who is filling the openings in the schedule and following up on past due patients? To think the practice can truly run efficiently without a business staff is an insult to the many business staff in dentistry who work diligently on the front lines and behind the scenes to make it happen!

As mentioned before, there's no one-size-fits-all in management. If you practice successfully in the frontdesklessness model, congratulations! Typically, however, there are breakdowns in communication and busy clinical staff must immediately return to the clinical area with little time to return calls, pull a chart, talk to an insurance company, or greet the next patient.

With this general formula in mind, you have the information you need to determine whether level revenues in your office for the past year or five years are a result of inadequate staffing.

If inadequate staffing is to blame, you'll notice three things will begin to happen:

1. Your accounts receivable will start to climb, which translates into more account statements to be generated and monitored and more work for just about everyone.

2. If your practice has a hygienist, you'll notice that the number of hygiene patients never goes up, even though the practice attracts thirty new patients each month. So non growth in the hygiene department is another indication that you're understaffed at the front desk. No one is concentrating on patient retention and calling past due preventive care patients. It is not uncommon for a practice to only be recalling twenty-five percent to forty percent of the patients in the central file.

3. The third thing you'll notice is that the morale in the office will

decline. When the front desk business staff start to show signs of overwhelm, the back office staff usually follow suit.

Clear Job Descriptions at the Desk

I believe in teamwork, but I also believe in clearly defined duties at the desk. It's helpful to all clinical people to know whom to go to at the front desk, whether they have a scheduling, financial, or insurance question.

I'm often asked whether it's wise to job share in the business office. At the front desk, a practice really needs continuity. If patients see a lot of job sharing in the business arena—that is, lots of different faces—it's confusing and disruptive. Also, there tend to be more breakdowns in communication that aren't conducive to practice growth. If, however, the two people job sharing in the business arena have exceptional communication with one another and they think alike and follow the same set of rules for practice systems, it's possible.

A Boat Can't Sail with Anchors in the Water

Who are your anchors? Take a snapshot of where your practice was five years ago. What did it look like? What does it look like today? Visualize what you'd like it to look like five years from now. How much revenue? How many people on the team? How large is the office?

Now think of each member of your staff as an individual and then as part of the team and answer these questions:

1. Does this person readily adapt to new technology and other advances affecting dentistry and dental practice management?
2. Does this person arrive on time, pulled together and ready to work?
3. Does the person do more than the basic expectations of the job, suggesting new ideas, and new ways of getting things done?
4. Does this person avoid uncharitable and unconstructive gossip about fellow staff members and patients?
5. Does the person often help out other team members overwhelmed by their responsibilities?

6. Is this person a positive voice for the office, one from whom you'd never hear self-defeating phrases like, "That'll never work," "We tried that once and it didn't work," "Our patients won't like that," or "We tried that in another office and it didn't work"?

Count your no's. Even one signals an improvement opportunity that requires counseling with the employee. More than one and certainly as many as five or more requires some serious rethinking about the role this person is playing in the business. You most likely have an anchor on your hands…someone you must ask to leave.

Bear in mind that keeping employees on staff because they are nice or because they are visible within the community costs the average dentist about $100,000 per year—on top of the employee's salary.

Sometimes people burn out in their position. Sometimes the practice is trying to move in a different direction that does not make that person happy anymore. You now have a responsibility to yourself, other members of the team, and your patients to take action. Try to mend the fence first rather than face the prospect of training a new employee.

Here's a sample discussion I might have with someone who's performance is indicating they're an anchor:

> *"Sue, you know how much I care about you. Last night I wrote down the many wonderful qualifications you have brought to my practice for the last eight years, the qualities in a dental assistant that I would have a hard time finding in another assistant if I were to ever lose you. While I was at it, I made a list of the three areas of frustration or resistance that are causing me stress. I made a decision last night, Sue. This was a business decision, not a personal decision. I have made a decision that I need one-hundred percent accountability and support of where I want this practice to be in five years. So I need your support, but I also want you to know that you are now on a thirty-day probation and you have thirty days to decide whether you want to go with the new system and the new ways of doing things, or whether you would be happy working somewhere else."*

If Sue doesn't improve, it's time to say, "Your letter of resignation will gladly be accepted in exchange for our letter of recommendation on all your good qualities so that you can work somewhere else."

Please Note
In order to dismiss an employee, you need signed reprimand forms for each misdeed.

Sample Reprimand Form

On _____[date]______, we discussed the following performance issue:

____

____

____

Employee check one:
❑ I agree.
❑ I disagree because

____

____

____

Employee Signature ______________________________
Employer Signature ______________________________
Date ___________________________

Give the employee a copy and keep a copy in their file. This is essential for eliminating any possibility of being accused of bias or impulsive decision making in your terminations.

CHAPTER 4

Scheduling Success!

EFFECTIVE SCHEDULING PRACTICES WILL MAKE OR BREAK YOUR DENtal practice, yet far too often when I visit a dental practice, I see treatment chairs that remain empty for too long during the day, reception rooms filled with patients looking impatiently at their watches. As if all that weren't enough, then I learn about office policies that discourage emergency patients and see appointment cards that are worded in such a way that they seem to be literally begging for a last minute cancellation or a no-show.

Every one of these practices and many more will cost you...big time. And not just in lost production. The practice will suffer on many levels: poor motivation, general confusion, excess paperwork and phone time, and missed lunch breaks.

Not the picture of a dental practice that's going to achieve breakthrough success, is it?

The very good thought, is that with a few simple changes and new disciplines, your practice can eliminate productivity-sapping time wasters—very quickly. Proper scheduling, good time management, effective handling of emergencies...these strategies and more will change your practice into a dynamic dental practice.

Let's begin with some simple time management strategies.

Being organized with a simple time management system makes life and work much more productive, and much easier. Put together a team of people who know how to manage time for maximum effectiveness and you'll see a happier, thriving, and far more productive dental office. This is because I've found time and again that a practice's profit margin is directly proportionate to the way the dental team manages its time.

It's really no wonder there are so many courses, books, and manuals today that are devoted to the topic of time management. The world is in fast forward at the same time all our To-Do lists and priorities are expanding. What do I do first? Then what? And then what? So many priorities vie for our time and attention that effective time management is a must.

Of course we each have the same twenty-four hours to spend each day. Many people try to save time, or borrow it for that matter. Time can only be spent. The trick to effective time management is to create a schedule that makes maximum use of each hour, and then to stick to it. With simple time management tips, you can start spending time more productively and when you do, more time becomes available for the things you must do but continually postpone. Time passes despite our pleas or prayers, but time management techniques enable us to control and maximize the time we do have.

Three Lists

The most powerful time management strategy is the simplest: create three lists at the end of each day for the following day. This only takes about five minutes a day but conserves many hours a week:

1. To Do. These are the things you want to do tomorrow. Those that are most urgent should be listed first and numbered in order of priority of importance.

2. To Call. These are the people you must call tomorrow to make things happen, or whose calls must be returned.

3. To Go. These are the errands you must run such as to the bank, insurance company, or lawyer's office.

Make your list, then close the door and go home.

Throughout the next day, mark off the items on each list as you complete them and don't end the day without doing one of two things: completing all the tasks on your lists or moving them to the following day's lists.

It's that simple.

We've all heard the saying, "If you want something done, take it to a busy person." The reason is that busy people are usually well organized, which enables them to get so much more done each day.

I've used this list system for years, and I find I accomplish much more with my time. The end of each day brings feelings of accomplishment and satisfaction, all while enabling me to complete more work each day. Sometimes I find that on a restless night if I get up and simply add whatever I'm concerned about to one of my lists, I sleep like a baby.

You can also expand this simple strategy to plan your time weekly. Make these week-long lists on Friday for the coming week.

Time-Tested Strategies

You, too, can accomplish more than you ever imagined if you write it down or enter it into your Palm Pilot and then go for it. The old saying "Plan your work, and then work your plan" is the secret of time management. Here are some time-honored strategies...

Set priorities for your work

Avoid the mistake in thinking that leads many people to operate as if a priority is what's on the top of the stack, or the person who shouts the loudest for attention, or the easiest jobs. You'll find that continually setting priorities this way does nothing to make you more effective and productive; it simply adds to your sense of being overwhelmed each day.

First, change your definition of a priority: a priority is a task with a deadline. Some examples:

- ✧ having all patient charts pulled and confirmed for the following day by 11:00 a.m.
- ✧ filling holes in the schedule the minute after one happens
- ✧ processing insurance forms immediately

- ✧ developing a marketing plan by the deadline set by the marketing company
- ✧ arranging for airline tickets to attend the ADA meeting before the best rates are gone
- ✧ sterilizing the instruments before they are needed in the next treatment room
- ✧ ordering supplies before they are completely exhausted
- ✧ getting the case back from the lab BEFORE the patient is in the dental chair for a cementation
- ✧ getting to the bank with the daily deposits before closing time
- ✧ registering for a course before it's sold out

Never put off today what can make tomorrow easier and less stressful.

> **Here's another tip:** rather than give in to the temptation to do the fun and easy things first, which only postpones the difficult work to a time in the day when you're not feeling particularly energetic or ready to handle a challenge, do the tough stuff first. Get it off your desk and off your mind as early in the day or week as you can.

Break large jobs down into smaller, more manageable ones

Remember the saying, "You can only eat an elephant one bite at a time." Start nibbling at a job and watch it disappear. Another saying comes into play here: "Well begun is half done." We waste so much energy procrastinating about a large or not terribly pleasant job yet, how many times have you found that once you got started, it wasn't so bad after all? That's because it's breaking your inertia to begin a task that can take the most energy and spirit. Begin the task, and more than half the time you'll find you misjudged the difficulty or overestimated the time you'll need to finish it.

Reward yourself when you meet an important goal or deadline
A healthy reward like flowers, a walk in the park, or even the (very occasional) chocolate treat will keep you inspired and motivated to reach for the next goal...and the next.

Avoid interruptions
In a busy dental practice, it's possible to be interrupted forty to sixty times a day. There's not much you can do to avoid these interruptions at the front desk where part of the job is being "interrupted" 100 to 150 times a day with telephone calls, patients coming and going, and the needs of the doctor and the rest of the staff. (One thing you can do, however: use written or computerized communication from the back office to the front desk, a strategy that has been proven to reduce front desk interruptions by as much as forty to fifty percent.)

Proper training is the first step to minimizing interruptions. The second is to stop and think, can I figure this out myself and does my doctor trust me to make decisions on my own that will improve efficiency and time management in everyday procedures?

Everyone should think before interrupting, "Can I figure this out or must I again ask someone?" Many times I've interviewed the staff privately to learn that in their practice they MUST ask the dentist everything because he or she demands this level of control!

Having well-trained, self-directed staff is the key to superior time management. In one client's office, the scheduling coordinator was not allowed to make scheduling decisions. She went to the treatment area a dozen times per day to ask the dentist if she could bring in an emergency, or schedule a patient in the opening for Tuesday? Hiring, training, and—this is key—trusting are the keys to effective delegation. To put the dental assistant in the position of having to ask the doctor, "Can I mix? Is this the right burr? Is this dry enough" not only wastes time but makes the staff look incompetent. Interruptions are truly the biggest source of time management problems.

Minimize unnecessary phone time
When it comes to interruptions during the business day, improper use of the phone is the biggest culprit. Not only does answering the phone take

you away from the task at hand, it usually demands some type of follow-up conversation or action involving yet another co-worker who's being taken away from yet another task. If you spent the time to add up the number of lost production hours caused by improper use of the phone, you'd be astonished by the number of dollars lost.

Save time on the phone by first making a list of the things you need to discuss before you pick up the phone to initiate a call. Avoid chit chat as much as possible, with the simple statement, "Let me just tell you quickly the reason for my call..."

When you're on the receiving end of a call, tell long-winded callers you have another call waiting. You might even consider starting the conversation with, "Oh Mary, I'm glad you caught me as I was just on my way to an important meeting" or, if you're making the call, "While my patient is getting numb, I want to spend a couple of minutes discussing Ms. Jones's periodontal progress."

Have firm policies about personal phone calls

Clear policies about personal calls can add hundreds of hours to the practice's daily production figures, which translates into tens of thousands of dollars each year, not to mention increasing the overall professionalism of the office. Consider that if seven people on staff receive three personal calls in a day, that amounts to twenty-one unnecessary interruptions for the desk staff. Even if each of these calls takes just three minutes, the office has lost about an hour of time for the day, four to five hours per week. That's approximately 225 hours per year! At an hourly production rate of $500 this is an annual loss of $112,500. When staff wonder why there is no money for raises, remind them that their daily habits can increase or decrease production even though it seems quite innocent to take or make a few calls per day.

The bottom line on personal calls is to start from the premise that they are generally not permitted. While some may be necessary, they must be kept very brief:

Yes: A child calling to ask what time Mom will be home.

No: A call from a sister or girlfriend to discuss what happened at the party last night, or plans for the weekend.

Yes: A dental assistant calling home to say she'll be a half hour late.
No: A scheduling coordinator calling a friend to ask advice about something.

Here's an example of language you might consider including in your employee handbook on the subject of personal calls:

> Personal calls tie-up phone lines and take time away from our patients. Every effort should be made to handle personal situations during non-working hours. However, we realize that employees must sometimes make and/or receive personal phone calls. Personal calls made or received during work hours must be kept very brief, and family and friends should be discouraged from calling during patient hours, except in the case of emergencies.

Most important, everyone on the staff—including the doctors—must abide by the policy. This is fair and sets the right example. It also makes it clear that policies are set in the interest of keeping the office at maximum productivity, and everyone has a role to play in that effort.
(For much more on setting and adhering to office policies, see Chapter 9.)

Important!
If state law allows a duty to be delegated to someone of a lesser salary, it should be. State dental practice acts should be reviewed to determine the maximum allowable use of expanded duty auxiliaries.

Files

The accountants and attorneys who serve your dental practice can tell you how long tax and business files must be retained. Your state's insurance commissioner can tell you how long insurance files must be kept. Your state's employment commission can provide a list of what records must be retained for past employees, present staff, and job applicants. Finally, you might decide to have a permanent file for records you will never discard, such as correspondence from the federal or state government on your practice's tax filing status, trademark documents, and the like. Patient records must be retained for seven years (adults) and up to the age of twenty-one for children patients. Because storage for these records requires so much space, micro-film or micro-fiche is best. For paperless offices, backing up on tapes or discs that are kept in safe storage for the standard number of years is required.

Once you know which files need to be retained and for how long, you can begin to clean house—or office! Discard any files the business simply does not need and organize the balance accordingly.

At the end of each calendar year, store business files that must be retained in an out of the way place. Keep these records (only for as long as they are required!) in file boxes with the year and contents clearly marked on the end of each box. This project usually takes place between the December holidays when the practice has down time. Some offices routinely schedule an end of the year organizational "party" on a particular day when the dentist and staff come in casually dressed and organize every inch of the office.

The business staff make room for the new general files for the upcoming year, the hygienists work on inactive recare patients and their treatment rooms, and the assistants completely organize the lab and the doctor's treatment rooms.

The dentist is in charge of his or her own desk and private office. Try placing a large towel on the top of your desk and empty drawers on the towel one at a time. It's amazing how much junk accumulates in one year that can be thrown away.

Imagine going to work on January 2 with everything completely organized! Now that's an end-of-year party that pays dividends for the remainder of the year. Some dentists and staff reading this say, "Oh my, we have never done this so it may take more than a day." Whatever it takes, make this an annual ritual. Watch your stress go down and your productivity go up. Bring in breakfast at 8:00 a. m. and plan your strategies for the day to optimize the hours there. Have lunch delivered and share your progress.

At the end of the day, have an informal celebration and go home happy rather than dreading the start of a new year totally disorganized.

Patient Scheduling

Now that you've eliminated both the obvious and hidden time wasters in your business day, your practice is on the road to maximizing the time available to treat patients and, more specifically, to generate revenue.

Because patients generate revenue—and everything else is overhead—it is not an exaggeration to say that nothing is more essential to the smooth, profitable operation of a dental practice than proper patient scheduling.

These are dynamic dentistry's Golden Rules of patient scheduling:

1. Every time you see an empty dental chair, you are temporarily unemployed.

2. When the patient's mouth closes, production stops.

3. No patient should ever leave the office without having made the next appointment.

The key to effective, productive scheduling is to have a patient being treated in each dental chair, each hour of each working day, with the exception of emergency flex time (for much more on scheduling emergency flex time, see page 126). Reread this sentence and focus on the phrase "being treated." This is what I mean when I say "Don't seat until you're ready to treat" because when a patient is sitting idly in a treatment room, not only is that patient either very anxious or very irritated about having his time wasted, the practice is not making money. A treatment chair in which a patient sits without being treated is therefore the same as an empty treatment chair!

We must also learn that the best time to schedule the next appointment is at the end of the present appointment, when the patient is in the office, thinking about their dental needs, not at home, distracted by fifty other priorities. (Anytime you hear the words "I'll call you," the practice is losing production!) So a patient should never leave without knowing when his next appointment is. If the patient cannot commit to an appointment for any reason, his name should be placed in the computer on the pending appointment list under the category of treatment needed. The scheduling coordinator can then contact him in the future. The pending list is a powerful way to boost production by enabling the scheduling coordinator to keep track of the people who don't schedule or call to cancel and don't reschedule. (You'll read much more on all these strategies throughout this chapter.)

Maximizing treatment time, keeping a constant flow of patients in treatment chairs, taking steps to eliminate cancellations and no-shows…all these patient scheduling strategies and more keep a high-performing scheduling coordinator—and the rest of the staff for that matter—sharply focused on scheduling dynamics within the practice. These are challenging tasks that require attention, discipline, and accountability.

State-of-the-Art Equipment

Under-equipping an office means having too little equipment or outdated equipment, including everything from an amalgamator and spittoon to the computers at the front desk. State-of-the-art technology in a dental office is not a luxury; it's a must.

Outdated equipment is costly because it slows down whoever must use it, and it sends a message to patients that the office doesn't invest in equipment that will provide the highest quality of care. In addition, old equipment breaks down and must be repaired, costing the practice twice: the money spent on the repair itself, as well as the lost productivity that results from not being able to treat patients, not to mention the phone calls and paperwork that finding a reliable repair service entails. This is why I call skimping on equipment false economy. It will only result in frustration, low morale, and lost production.

And the same piece of equipment should NEVER be shared between treatment rooms. All treatment rooms must be adequately equipped with similar setups. With all the current health risks faced by patient and clinical staff alike, today more than ever, we must be certain that each treatment room is adequately equipped with properly sterilized instruments.

Good Delegation

Proper delegation is an essential time management skill and a bit of an art because it involves successful communication and persuasion. Yet, anyone—especially professionals like dentists who generate revenue only when they're delivering their expertise and not when they're handling administrative details—who knows how to delegate effectively enjoys the highest productivity and the lowest stress.

The first rule of successful delegation is that delegation isn't dumping, that is handing someone a stack of paper and quickly walking away with a sense of relief. Successful delegating includes:

- ✧ Clear and specific instructions. Don't expect someone to read your mind. Be clear about what needs to be done and by when. If you can provide written in addition to verbal guidelines, all the better.
- ✧ Encouragement to use personal knowledge and skills. Sometimes, you need someone to follow directions to a T, and when this is the case, you must make it clear that there can be no deviation from the instructions you've provided. However, as often as possible, you should encourage people to make suggestions for improvement on a process or task you've delegated to them. Explain that you're open to their feedback and ideas for improvement, and set a tone for accepting and using positive, constructive feedback by listening to ideas and using the best of them.
- ✧ Expressions of confidence. When you hand over a task, tell the person you know they can do it, and then make it clear through your actions that you really mean it. Step away from the task and let the person get it done for you.
- ✧ A reasonable deadline. It's unfair to delegate a task with an impossible deadline attached, especially if the person accepting the job has little or no experience in the area. Be certain to set a reasonable deadline for getting the job done that also enables

you to provide the person with feedback and still gives him sufficient time to make adjustments as needed before the final deadline.

✧ Finding the right person for the task. People do much better jobs if they like what they're doing. Before delegating a job, spend some time thinking about who would enjoy the task and/or whose talents would be best used on this particular job.

✧ Appreciation. Staff members should be complimented for accepting delegated tasks and praised when they perform well.

Here's an example of the impact successful delegation can have on production: a large number of dentists are still doing prophys. They say, "If I don't do prophys about fifty hours a month, I won't be busy," yet this statement has been proven wrong time and again. When the hygienist sees all the prophys and sets the stage for a high percentage of case acceptance in the process, the doctor's fifty hours are spent doing restorative dentistry instead of work that can be delegated. I have seen dozens of offices double their production with this simple change that involves effective delegation. Smart business, powerful bottom line results!

High Energy

I've met dentists who like to anesthetize a patient, then leave to read the newspaper and have a cup of coffee. These are the same dentists who complain about low production!

In contrast, successful businesses of all kinds approach the day with velocity, energy, and intensity. They move quickly, provide excellent service, and get out on time for lunch and at the end of the day. Make sure your practice is among them by doing all you can to eliminate time-wasting habits and tasks and hiring people with energy and excitement for the practice of dentistry.

Beware of dental team players who think small, often the culprit behind low motivation and energy levels in an office. They may be fixed on a mental picture of a $40,000 monthly production figure, and not a penny more.

Some of these team members may say things like: "We always have a bad December. People are saving their money for the holidays, you know," or "The practice will never do more than $25,000 a month as we're rural." In fact, December should be a banner month because patients are likely to use that time to take advantage of the last of the year's insurance coverage. And some of the more successful practices I know are rural. Not surprisingly, practices can and often do double their production when they double their goals.

We become what we think—for better or worse. In the words of Henry Ford, "Whether you think you can or you think you can't, you're right."

Appointment Control

Computerized scheduling has become a godsend to dentistry when as recently as the early '90s, dentists and staff were still struggling to accept this new model of scheduling. Today, we wonder how the office survived without it. Business staff were afraid the computer would "eat" the schedule, and "What if we have a power failure; we can lose everything!"

Some of the older dentists resisted the change, often because they felt incapable of accessing the schedule when they saw patients on the weekend. It was not unheard of for older business staff to resign or retire rather than give up their security of the paper appointment books. Imagine! Now, there isn't—or shouldn't be!—a practice out there that operates without computerized scheduling. With back-up tapes and power surge/failure and virus protections built in, offices are much more at ease with the transition.

All computer schedules have color coding and block scheduling capabilities. The Pending Appointment Systems of all schedulers have improved over the years so that patients who have not scheduled in advance or who cancel and don't reschedule can be easily tracked.

In color coding or block scheduling, determine how many major procedures are needed to reach a certain production goal such as crown and bridge in a general practice, bandings in Ortho, surgery or implant dentistry in Perio, etc. Block out a particular number of appointment blocks by a specific color (yellow) and reserve it for just those appointments. Next determine a color for basic restorative dentistry (blue), and the amount of time units for these procedures each day in column one (primary treatment).

Set aside time in the schedule for new patient interviews, consultations, emergencies, staff meetings, etc. Green is the color used in many practices for down time or a time for the assistant to be doing other important duties such as ordering supplies while the dentist does a consultation. Red is the color most often used for minor surgeries or extractions.

Hopefully, if your practice is not color coding and block scheduling, the above ideas will assist you in going this route. Otherwise, your production will remain below par, you will constantly work into lunch and home time, and you will have no place to put larger case dentistry because you'll be cluttering the schedule with daily non-productive procedures.

Patients who have to wait to start major treatment plans get buyer's remorse or go somewhere else once their mind is made up to have the total care started and finished by a particular time. If the office tells them their treatment can begin the next month, but they have a twentieth class reunion or other important event such as a wedding, they'll find a practice with blocked time that gets the major treatment finished in time.

We have to learn to engineer and color code/block schedule rather than just throw these names anywhere just to fill up space.

The Dental Assistant and the Initial Patient Interview—A Great Time Saver

People who call the office as non-emergency new patients should be seen within three or four days. Handled properly, the initial patient interview is an opportunity to save time while building a strong relationship between the patient and the practice. Since dental assistants are permitted to interview patients in most states, they can assist the doctor on the patient's first visit.

Patients readily accept staff when doctors trust the staff and show that trust in ways that are visible and meaningful to patients. A simple introduction of the dental assistant to the patient made by the doctor helps to set the stage for the patient feeling comfortable and confident in the practice.

> **Staff live up to the level of trust their dentist has in their ability**
> If the dentist is not a delegater and believes he is the only person who can perform these interviews, staff will soon begin to hesitate, ques-

tion their own judgment, and show a lack of initiative. Delegation is an essential and valuable way in which the dentist shows faith in staff. This communicates to staff and ultimately to patients. And the results are nothing short of amazing. Higher morale, higher patient retention, more referrals, higher productivity…and a more pleasant work place in the bargain!

Follow this example of a well-handled initial patient interview:

The doctor walks into the treatment room with the dental assistant, introduces himself or herself, and then says, "This is Sherry, my new patient coordinator. I've asked her to spend some time with you now. She will be asking some very important questions, taking the necessary x-rays, and getting other pertinent data. As soon as she is finished, I'll be back for a thorough examination." The doctor then returns to work in another treatment room.

Sherry sits in the doctor's chair with the chart in clear view with an attitude of concern and interest. Her goal is to gather the needed information in a way that makes the new patient feel as if he is the only one being treated that day.

Sherry begins the interview with two essential questions, noting the patient's answers on the chart or in the computer. The first one is "Mr. Stephens, before we do anything else, tell me how you feel about keeping your natural teeth for a lifetime." We can talk to patients endlessly about what they need, but people only buy what they want. Your goal as the new patient coordinator is to guide the patients to want what they need.

Mr. Stephens may say, "Well, my parents both lost their teeth around age thirty-five. I am now thirty-three. I guess it's about time for me to lose mine." Or he may say, "My parents both lost their teeth at an early age, and I will do everything I can to keep mine."

The second question Sherry asks is, "Is there anything about your teeth or smile you don't like?" Many people don't like their smiles and would like to change them.

The strategy here is simple: If patients first hear their dental needs identified by the dentist, they think "money." But when staff members have asked positive questions that lead into a dental discussion and the doctor then reinforces the need, the patients think "concern."

Important!
A point to keep in mind when interviewing new patients is that staff members can never diagnose; only doctors can. But staff members can ask questions that plant positive seeds of need.

Next, Sherry reviews the health questions with the patient and marks in red pencil any medical problems that have been identified. She enters these medical notes into the computer, then places red medic alert tape on the outside of the patient's chart for instant referral to the medical problem. She then does the blood pressure screening and recording and charts the existing restorations.

Important!
When the entire staff is focused on the patient's complete health, it sends an important message that the practice is, in fact, interested in the patient's total health, not just their teeth.

In charting existing restorations in gray lead pencil on the paper clinical record or entering it into the computerized chart, Sherry asks questions such as, "Has anyone ever mentioned replacing this lower first molar, Mr. Stephens?" or "Does the edge of this fractured tooth bother you?"

Because Sherry charts the existing restorations, the dentist will have before-and-after visual aids in the treatment room.

When the doctor walks into the treatment room for the complete examination, everything is organized and ready. The clinical record should be placed for the doctor's review. The patient's likes and dislikes, feelings about his other teeth, blood pressure, medical information, and charting can be reviewed by the doctor.

The dentist then performs a soft tissue exam, oral cancer screening, occlusal evaluation, and spot periodontal probing. Using simple terminology ("chewing surface," "cheek side," "tongue side," "front" and "back") so the patient understands what's being said, the doctor calls off exactly what Mr. Stephens needs on teeth 1 through 32.

> Next, Sherry reads back the information to ensure it is charted or entered into the computer correctly. This also serves as double reinforcement for the patient. On smaller treatment plans, the case discussion should be held chairside rather than with a full consultation. On larger cases, the full consultation with digital photos, models, x-rays, and a custom designed treatment plan is a necessity.

It's easy to see how having a skilled dental assistant conduct three-fourths of the communication and data collection on the initial interview can free up hundreds of hours per year of the doctor's time and build a strong total practice relationship with the patient in the process...a powerful win-win! With thirty-five new patients per month, thirty of them adults, this amounts to 360 hours a year. Three-fourths of this time is a 270 hours savings of time. At $500 per hour, this is a production increase of $135,000 annually.

The standard objection to this strategy is that the dentist must develop rapport with his or her patients. Rapport is essential; however, there are a number of ways to build it. Having the dental assistant conduct this interview helps a patient develop rapport with the entire practice while freeing up forty to forty-five minutes of the dentist's time.

Some courses actually recommend that the dentist spend ninety minutes in the new patient examination because they can't be thorough in less time. In that case, every patient they see for ninety minutes better need a full mouth reconstruction to compensate for the forty-five hours of the dentist's time used monthly in conducting this interview.

Despite all this, I've often heard staff members object to having the dental assistant conduct this interview, saying instead that it's best done by a hygienist since patients want their teeth cleaned on the first appointment. And indeed this is often the case. The trouble is that the scheduling coordinator has no way of knowing how much time to schedule for the cleaning in these instances, since the patient is brand new to the practice. A better strategy is to tell the new patient what the initial visit will entail, and then explain, "The doctor's exam will tell us the amount of time our hygienist will need with you for your first preventive care appointment."

On rare occasions, a new patient might say, "I'm in a wedding in ten days, and I thought I should get my teeth cleaned." Try to accommodate these patients by dovetailing the appointments, scheduling thirty minutes with the New Patient Coordinator (second dental assistant) and thirty minutes with the hygienist. If this scheduling strategy isn't feasible, the hygienist may see a few new patients.

A Hygienist/Assistant Team

The wave of the future for more efficient scheduling in the hygiene department is assisted hygiene, in which a hygienist has her own designated full-time assistant working out of two treatment rooms. Imagine for a minute how many dentists would become burned out and unproductive if they were placed in a situation in which they had one treatment chair, no assistant, and no flexibility. In other words, they'd have a schedule to adhere to but they'd also have two other people (the patient and the person doing their examination) who could make or break their time management.

Assisted hygiene is not new. In the eighties it was called accelerated hygiene, and the program was fraught with problems. It became an assembly line operation of double booking patients with no clear job description for a poorly trained support staff, including the scheduler and the assistant who was helping in between assisting for the dentist. Thus, the best concept for the future of dentistry developed a bad reputation and is still looked upon by some people today with disdain and concern.

There are several reasons for this concern:

1) Some hygienists fear that allowing the smart and well-trained dental assistants of today to have more direct patient care is the first step in doing away with the hygienist position. That, of course, will never happen as the hygiene department and the hygienist are the backbone of the practice. Studies prove time and again that the healthier the hygiene department, the stronger and more profitable the practice.

2) Some hygienists and dentists have expressed fear that the patient may feel "passed off" in this arrangement. Remember, the patient accepts what the office accepts! Dynamic practices have positive ideas about change and introducing new concepts to their patients. Hygienists within these

practices introduce assisted hygiene by saying, "Mrs. Harris, please meet Tara, my assistant. Today you will be treated royally by not just one member of our team but both of us." Of course having the right assistant is a key factor, according to my friend Anastasia Turchetta, RDH, from North Carolina who teaches assisted hygiene and has practiced this model since 1998. Personalities must blend, work ethics must be similar, and most important, both team members should value their own and the other's contribution to this model of care.

3) Some hygienists fear they may develop a problem like carpal tunnel syndrome from seeing thirteen to fourteen patients per day. For many hygienists, this is a top concern. Now, after doing assisted hygiene for months or years, many hygienists say, "I fought the concept even though we were losing over 200 patients per month in hygiene due to the fact we could not find a second hygienist in our small town. We had two hygiene chairs and tried assisted hygiene, and now I go home happy tired rather than stressed-out tired" or "I call us the Dynamic Duo. I would never want to work solo hygiene again. With my assistant doing all the peripheral duties, I can concentrate on my patients and my wrists and hands feel better on this schedule than they ever did doing everything myself." Still others have said, "I wish I had practiced this way for the past ten years. I can't imagine doing it any other way."

4) Hygienists wonder whether their salary will increase if they see more patients. Assistants wonder, "Will I make less assisting in the hygiene department versus assisting the dentist?" In the solo hygiene scenario, the salary for the hygienist is usually thirty to thirty-five percent of their production without the exams, twenty-five percent if exams are counted as hygiene production. In the assisted hygiene model, I encourage my clients to take the combined hygienist and assistant salaries for those two chairs and pay the assistant the same hourly as if they assisted in any position in the office based on attitude, performance, and results. Pay the hygienist (minus her assistant's salary) thirty percent of his or her combined production, or pay the hygienist a certain dollar amount for each patient seen beyond the normal eight or nine in solo hygiene. At $10 per patient extra from an additional six patients a day (from eight to four-

teen), this is a $60 per day bonus or an additional $11,520 per year for seeing more patients in the assisted hygiene model. The assistant is on the team incentive plan; the hygienist is salaried, plus her own $10 per patient extra; therefore, the hygienist is not on the team incentive plan as her commission plus salary is an incentive-based pay model.

The optimum schedule for assisted hygiene is simple. Here's an example: one patient is in chair one at 8:00 a.m. and a second patient is in chair two at 8:10 a.m. A third is in chair one at 8:50 a.m. and a fourth is in chair two at 9:00 a.m. This zig-zag schedule allows for fifty minutes of chair time for each adult patient with the assistant seeing the patient for the first ten minutes to seat, update their personal and health history, (Has the patient changed his mailing address, home, or work telephone numbers? Jobs or insurance carriers? What is his e-mail address for the practice's e-newsletter and appointment confirmations that the practice will be sending via e-mail soon? Is the patient taking any new medications?) The assistant also does the blood pressure screening and recording. She takes x-rays as indicated or prescribed.

The next thirty minutes is the hygiene time for scaling, educating, and "talking dentistry." The last ten minutes is dental assistant time for coronal polishing (in some states), oral hygiene instructions, standing in the exam, charting needed treatment, pre-appointing the next recare visit appointment (also pre-appointing operative if this is not done at the front desk at check out), and tearing down and re-setting the treatment room.

In this model, if the average hygiene fee is $105 without bitewing x-rays and $140 with them. Six patients that day needed bite-wings, two quadrant scales at $160, and five patients were regular recare visits (adults). All together, this hygienist/assistant team produced $1,685 in one day. For an eight hour day, the hygienist in this model makes approximately $48 per hour while the assistant makes about $15/hour. If this sounds intriguing and fair, you are a good candidate for this model. (The hygienist's and assistant's combined compensation is 29.9 percent of their production that day.)

Some staff feel they should be paid by educational background, longevity in the practice or the profession, etc. However, compensation can only come from attitudes, performance, and results. You can have the most highly skilled, highly educated, or trained staff in dentistry, but if they have "stinkin thinkin" as motivational speaker and author Zig Ziglar calls it, they are hurting your practice. Not accepting new models of care as they come along in my opinion falls into this category of "thinkin."

CHAPTER 5

Reducing No-Shows and Broken Appointments

WELCOME TO THE WORLD OF THE FULL APPOINTMENT SCHEDULE! A world in which patients make appointments...and consistently keep them. A world where failed or changed appointments are the rare exception and occur for only the most honest reasons, and no one even knows how to spell n-o s-h-o-w.

This is the dynamic dentistry world of scheduling-savvy. And it can be yours, with a few simple—yes, simple—changes. An average dental practice can be fifteen to thirty percent more productive if it eliminates the holes in doctors' and hygienists' schedules caused by broken appointments and no shows. Translate that into dollars, and it means that these scheduling problems are costing the practice something on the order of $100,000 to $200,00 or more annually! And, it's unnecessary!

A broken appointment is a loss to three people: the patient who missed the valuable time, another patient who could have used the valuable time, and the doctor who was fully staffed and prepared for the visit.

In fact, one broken hygiene appointment daily is a loss of $20,000 to $25,000 annually if the practice's average recare fee is $100 to $125 per patient visit. Hygiene is typically one-third of total volume, which means the dentist loses another $60,000 to $75,000 in restorative dentistry in the mouths of the patients who were not there as scheduled. If the staff ever wonders why there's no money for raises, this could be a key reason! Zero defects in the schedule should be every member of the team's goal.

Causes of Broken Appointments

Attitude. Let's start with attitude. It may surprise you to learn that reducing no-shows and broken appointments is mostly a matter of attitude and high quality communication. That's right. Fixing these vexing, production-sapping schedule problems is more a matter of the staff's attitude and the quality of the communication with patients about them than anything else.

In some offices, staff members accept a patient's excuses for changing and breaking appointments in a way that actually encourages them. The truth is, because they haven't scheduled what I call "organizational time"—time to complete routine behind-the-scenes duties such as collection calls, insurance follow up, confirmation calls, etc.—they subconsciously welcome these breaks in appointments as a way to catch up on busy work. Patients pick up on this attitude and don't take appointment times seriously. They fail or change appointments at the last minute for the slightest reason...again, largely because the staff makes it so easy to do so! They reschedule, filling up another appointment in the future, often during prime time hours, preventing another patient from being scheduled at that time. They may very well cancel or no-show again, leaving a prime time slot wide open and unproductive. Meanwhile, the honest patient who wanted that prime time slot got stuck coming in at 2:30. And on and on.

I've seen firsthand, though, how offices adopt "organizational time" and magically seem to have fewer holes in their schedules while the paperwork and other busy work gets done. This is because the staff in these offices have the time to devote their full attention to busy work during this time, and can also devote their full attention to patient handling and care during treatment hours. They no longer welcome schedule gaps, and make it clear to patients that because they take a scheduled appointment seriously, patients should too.

Broken appointments actually start chairside when the patients pick up on the dentist and clinical staff's value of the appointment time. If an office keeps the patient waiting more than ten minutes, patients assume being time-conscious is not a priority in this practice. The communication chairside must also be very positive. If the hygienist or hygiene assistant asks, "Mr. Bailey, would you like to make your next 'cleaning' appointment?" the patient is likely to respond with, "Oh, I have no idea what I'm doing in six days, much less six months." If the response back is, "Well, let's just go ahead and make the appointment for six months but when you get your card in the mail, if it isn't a good time you an always change it," these practices shouldn't wonder why they have eight broken appointments or no-shows a week while other practices have eight per month!

First of all, never refer to the preventive care appointment as the "cleaning," "recall," or "check-up." Each of these terms suggests these appointments are unimportant. "I can clean my own teeth. We recall broken appliances and faulty cars, and I only need a check-up if I have a problem!" is the patient's mental response.

Two of the most effective ways to reduce broken appointments and no-shows are:

1. Never invite patients to change their appointments for any reason, and
2. Don't ask if a patient wants to make an appointment for the next visit, but rather explain, "Mr. Bailey, if this time of day is good for you, I'd like to go ahead and reserve the same time of day, same day of the week in six months." If Mr. Bailey says, "I don't know what I'll be doing in six days much less six months," respond with, "Mr. Bailey, if you choose your reserved time now, you'll have a choice of appointment times. However, I do leave one appointment per day open for the small percentage of my patients who can't preschedule. If you don't appoint now, someone will call to schedule you in five months at which time you'll have to take one of those left-over appointments or risk not getting back into my schedule at

all." (No one likes leftovers and by sounding busy and in demand, the hygienist becomes busier and in high demand.)

Discouraging broken appointments or last-minute changes is a bit of an art and a skill that can be developed. Step one is to learn how to determine the patient's reasons for wanting to move the appointment, and then how to react accordingly.

Most patients with worthwhile reasons call early in the morning and start the conversation with an apology: "I'm so sorry I must change my appointment today, but my baby was up all night with an earache and her doctor's appointment is the same time as my dental appointment."

In handling this situation, the scheduling coordinator should say, "I understand completely, Mrs. White. Rather than take up your time now, I'll make a note to call you before 5:00 this afternoon to reschedule your appointment. Plus, I'll want to know that the baby's okay!" This shows true concern, not only for the patient but for her child as well.

On the other hand, you'll want to change your strategy if a patient calls with a feeble excuse like, "I didn't know it would be a sunny day, and I've decided to go to play golf."

If a patient places greater importance on golf or a hair appointment than a dental appointment, make rescheduling difficult:

- ✧ Sound disappointed, yet friendly. Don't immediately say things like, "That's okay" or "No problem" because the truth is, it's not really okay, and it is a problem!

- ✧ When rescheduling, don't offer the next available time or a prime time appointment. Instead, make rescheduling difficult in cases where the patient offers a feeble excuse by saying, "Oh, I'm sorry you and the children can't come in tomorrow to see our hygienist. It will be weeks before I can reserve three appointments together again." When rescheduling is not easy, the caller often decides it's more trouble to reschedule than to keep the appointment.

A special note on family appointments: If an entire family had a total of four hours of appointments and a parent is trying to reschedule, you might want to say, "Mrs. Brown, I'm so sorry you can't keep these appointments since we usually, just for this reason, don't grant multiple family appointments. In the future, I'm sure you'll understand why we can no longer see your family at one time and will have to schedule their appointments one at a time."

In my seminars, I encourage dentists to go across the parking lot and borrow a phone, disguise their voice, and pretend they are changing or breaking their largest appointment tomorrow to see what type of response their scheduling coordinator provides. If they sense relief in the person's voice, they can rest assured patients believe that open time makes the staff happy and they are doing you a favor! If the doctor receives a neutral response, again this is a negative sign that it is no big deal to cancel on short notice, and such cancellations will increase. If, however, the scheduling coordinator has had proper training and has the tone of friendly disappointment, repeat broken appointment offenders will not be the order of the day. I found that when I showed disappointment and made rescheduling difficult, I could talk more than sixty percent of the feeble excuse patients into keeping their appointments.

- ✧ When scheduling a patient for the next appointment, stress the importance of that visit, such as, "Your endodontic treatment was completed today. For best results, it is very important to go back to your referring dentist for the custom designed crown to preserve your investment here" or "You should have no problems with your temporary crown. However, it is important that you return in three weeks as scheduled." Many patients feel they can postpone treatment if they are not having a problem.

- ✧ Try saying, "I'm sorry you can't keep that appointment tomorrow with Susan, our hygienist. Her next available time is in three months." The usual response is, "Oh, in that case, I'd better keep it."

- ✧ Offer a creative option. I would offer to send a cab for people who had a two-hour crown and bridge appointment and attempted to cancel or postpone due to a car problem. I must have offered thirty taxies during my last year at the desk, but no one ever took me up on it. They always said, "Oh, I bet my neighbor, or the secretary at the next desk, will loan me their car."

✧ Finally, train the entire staff to avoid using the word "cancellation" because you don't want patients to know the practice ever has any such thing. Call them "schedule changes." If a patient must be moved forward to fill space tomorrow, say "We have a change in our schedule tomorrow at 3:00. Would you like to come in then?" If the word "cancellation" is used, the patient feels second best.

Lack of urgency. Consider the hygienist who says goodbye to a patient with these words: "Tom, it was great seeing you today. Say 'Hi' to Mary and the kids for me, and have fun on your golf tour!"

What a missed opportunity to provide the patient with a reason to return!

Note now the difference between this social approach and that of the hygienist who says, "Tom, it was great seeing you today. I'm glad you're doing so much better on your home care. Your gums are looking much less inflamed, which was our main goal. However, I'm still concerned about the inflammation on the lower left side of your mouth. We still have some work to do to get that under control. So keep at it, but that's the area I'm going to examine first when you're back in three months. Say 'Hi' to Mary and the kids for me, and have fun on your golf tour!"

Now Tom has a clear sense of urgency about keeping his next appointment. A reason to return will eliminate fifty percent or more of the openings in your schedule.

Misguided communication. A good example of this is the appointment card with the statement at the bottom that reads, "If unable to keep this appointment, kindly give us a twenty-four hours notice."

This statement sends a clear message that broken appointments are just fine as long as you tell us the day before!

Replace that message with this one: "This time has been reserved just [or specifically] for you. Please consider this card your confirmation." By handing out this appointment card, you make it crystal clear that not only do you expect the patient to show up on time for the appointment, you've already confirmed it. That sends a powerful message about what it means to do business with this dental practice by saying: "We treat our patients with the same seriousness and attention to detail that we treat our scheduling policies."

Playful recare cards. I prefer higher end recare cards, but there are more playful ones available. Choose those that match the needs of your particular demographics/market. If your practice is less interested in high end dentistry, than playful, less serious cards that feature cartoon characters may work for you.

Alternatively, if your patients are more likely to respond positively to cards depicting more serious, less playful graphics, consider postcards that depict a photograph of your beautiful reception area with the modern artwork turned into a postcard. This is a great option because it connects patients back to your office. If you are into cosmetic dentistry, use a postcard with a before and after photo of cosmetic dentistry and teeth whitening.

An unmotivated team. Another reason for broken appointments and open time in dentistry is a staff person who has the idea that they will make the same amount of money no matter how hard they work or how many patients are seen. Staff salaries are guaranteed. For this and other reasons, I highly recommend an incentive bonus plan. I remember loving them as an employee, and as an employer, I love them even more. Provide incentives based on production and collection levels, case acceptance, new patient numbers, hygiene department increases, patient satisfaction cards, or any other measure that helps to drive the business forward and upward.

There are hundreds of possible incentive formulas and program structures to provide both individual and team incentives that really work to motivate the group, and each individual in it. Create a program that will be effective in your unique practice.

As an added bonus, team incentives inspire staff to work together and build a sense of teamwork, healthy competition, and fun.

For more information on incentive bonus plans, including downloadable sample plans, visit my website at www.dentalmanagementU.com.

Filling Non-Prime Time Appointments

Every scheduling coordinator faces the challenge of filling non-prime time appointments. Some offices have two or three openings a day in non-prime time hours and they feel there's just no way to fill them, even though they're scheduled in prime time four months out. In these offices, the patients are controlling the schedule.

Here's a better way: Simply offer non-prime time hours to patients. What do I mean? Many times the prime time appointments are filled up first because that's what the scheduling coordinator offers the patient. Instead, suggest a non-prime time appointment first. Then, if the patient can't make any of those, consider a prime time appointment.

In my experience, patients take what you offer nine times out of ten. So offer them the two most difficult appointments to fill and break the habit of giving away the appointments that are easiest to fill. To illustrate this point, I often quote one of my former consultants, Char Sweeney from Michigan. "In the front row of a lecture, I pick an office with eight to ten people and playfully tell them I'm going out to pick up lunch for everyone in the front row. I tell them they have a choice of pizza or a turkey sandwich and go down the row asking which they prefer. Rarely does anyone break the cycle by saying, 'I really don't care for either, can you get me a salad instead?'" This proves that suggestive selling works even in offering non-prime time appointments.

If the scheduling coordinator says, "Dr. Wilson can see you on the fourteenth at eleven or on the sixteenth at ten," Patients will almost always choose one of the two. When the scheduling coordinator asks, "When would you like to come in?" the patient has the power to determine the schedule and they sense that appointments aren't scarce or sacred. The result: broken appointments and no-shows! In addition, prime time is filled months in advance and there are openings all week in non-prime time—the most difficult to fill!

Filler Appointments

Another reason broken or cancelled appointments cost a practice fifteen to thirty percent of its potential production each year is that there is no system for filling these holes the minute they occur.

Here's a better strategy: the pending list.

Using this strategy, a superior scheduling coordinator who gets a call changing the schedule immediately goes to work to remedy the open time. The doctor's or hygienist's problem is solved before he or she even knew there was one.

A pending appointment list, a list of patients who did not schedule or scheduled then changed the appointment, serves four valuable purposes:

1. It adds thousands of dollars to the office's monthly production.
2. Patients will stop falling through the cracks of the appointment schedule.
3. The stored information can be used to fill holes in the schedule the moment they happen. You've got an immediate source of names, numbers, and treatments to fill the hole in the schedule within five minutes of an opening taking place.
4. A dental practice can be held legally responsible for "lost patients." This recorded and stored information showing three attempts were made to reschedule is a big plus in the office's favor in the event of a "supervised neglect" case.

Your pending list should have six categories (specialists will differ):

1. Crown and bridge/veneers
2. Endodontic treatments
3. Simple restorations
4. Inlays and onlays
5. Recares
6. Miscellaneous

Remember dynamic dentistry's Golden Rule: "No patient should ever leave the office without having made the next appointment." If the patient's name does not go onto the main schedule, it should be entered into the computerized pending list under the type of treatment needed with the telephone number, treatment code, and length of treatment chair time needed.

A good scheduling coordinator will not leave the office for the day if there are holes in the next day's schedule.

With a computerized pending list organized by the type of treatment needed, the scheduling coordinator is able to push a button and see a screen full of single unit crowns, for instance, that are needed but haven't been scheduled.

Important!
When there is a gap in the schedule, never move an already scheduled patient into that time slot. This is a bad habit that not only creates havoc in your schedule, it strains patient relationships and sends the wrong message to patients who will begin to think that all appointments are merely the starting point for endless changes and reschedulings. Better to set the example—through your actions—that an appointment is an appointment. Use your pending list to fill gaps instead.

Rainy Day Call List

Consider creating something I call a "Rainy Day Call List," a list of people you know who are likely to be available in inclement weather, when others are just as likely to cancel due to the weather. Who's generally available when it rains? People who work outdoors like brick layers and construction workers, as well as people with outdoor hobbies like golfing. Call these people and check for their availability when others cancel due to poor weather.

I developed this strategy in 1977 while working for Dr. Richard S. Wilson of Richmond, Virginia, my last employer before starting my company full time in 1980. When I drove to the office with the windshield wipers going full speed, I knew many of the patients who loved Dr. Wilson's practice but feared driving in bad weather would become broken appointments that day. Sure enough, soon after I arrived at the office, I started to get the calls. "Oh, it's so bad outside and I don't drive when it rains hard. The James River may flood and I would not be able to get back home!" I responded with, "I know it's really bad as I just drove from Chester and I would not want you out there in this rain. Let's give you another appointment." This was the only time I was accommodating when confronted with a broken appointment that I expected. Fortunately, I had begun creating a Rainy Day Call List, and I immediately went to it and called those folks who could come on a rainy day! It worked like magic!

Short Notice (Special) Call List

If patients live or work within a two-mile radius of the office, consider not reappointing them before they leave the office. You might instead say, "Doris, since you work right next door, may I put you on my "special call list" and call you on short notice when a prime time appointment becomes available?" (not "…when I have a cancellation). You may find many patients saying they enjoy being considered "special" and having the freedom to decide on a given day whether they can come in, rather than having to tie up their own schedule in advance.

This is the type of creative thinking that enables you to fill in last minute openings and no shows…and add dramatically to your production.

> What is your doctor's ideal day, his or her most productive hours? Every scheduling coordinator should know the answer to this question. When is your doctor at his or her peak performance? Some doctors are not morning people, and yet the scheduling coordinator puts all their major treatment early in the morning. Some doctors don't reach their energy peak until after lunch. Make this determination, and factor it into the design of the day.

Lunch Is a Must!

Avoid scheduling the last half hour before lunch because this practice will invariably result in missed lunches or seriously abbreviated lunches for just about everyone at one point or another. Of course, this will also cause high levels of stress, low production (because happy people out-produce unhappy people), and eventually staff turnover. All that from a scheduling policy? You bet.

I want you to start enjoying the half hour before lunch as lag time in which you tear down, set up, and do whatever else is needed to get ready for the afternoon. Dentists need this time to return phone calls from the morning, work on treatment plans, or do lab work. Hygienists and dental assistants use this time for restocking their work areas and organizing their upcoming afternoon. They can also call patients who missed appointments or do chart audits for tomorrow's patients. Business staff use this time to tie up loose ends, work on accounting, return calls, and organize the balance of their day.

No one leaves until five minutes before the lunch hour officially begins so that they are back five minutes before it's officially over. Everyone teams up to help one another during this half hour. Then, they take a full, relaxing lunch break and return refreshed and ready for the rest of the day.

Here's what happens in the office in which lunch is frequently missed or shortened: staff members who actually get to take lunch sort of straggle back, the afternoon starts twenty minutes late, and everyone ends up working an extra hour every evening, which of course involves paying for overtime hours for many offices.

Change the way in which the day is scheduled to add a half hour of lag time (no appointments!) right before a scheduled lunch hour, incorporate better time management, eliminate wasted chair time, and watch attitudes improve...and production soar.

Finally...

The question invariably comes up in my seminars: Should we devote the time to make confirmation calls? My answer: maybe. They are not always effective.

First, in dynamic dentistry, we don't make "confirmation calls"; we make "courtesy calls." There's all the difference in the world between the two. A confirmation call suggests that the appointment hasn't already been confirmed (which of course it has since your appointment card says so!). Second, you don't call to remind your patient about an appointment because you run the risk of making the patient feel absentminded or irresponsible.

Here's a better approach. First, always have the scheduling coordinator make these calls, never the hygienist or anyone else for that matter. Appointments are the province of the scheduling coordinator who has ultimate responsibility for the quality and completeness of the schedule, and it is he or she who should take care that these calls are made and handled properly.

The scheduling coordinator should call one or two days in advance and say, "Hello, Mrs. Johnson. It's Linda at Dr. Wilson's office. This is your courtesy call to let you know we're looking forward to seeing you tomorrow at 11:00." The message is entirely different. The call isn't to remind the patient on the assumption that she has forgotten, but rather to say, "We're all looking forward to seeing you!" It makes the patient feel special, and that's a patient that will show up for the appointment with a smile.

A common question is if the patient isn't home and the scheduling coordinator reaches a recorded message, what should they do? Leave the following message: "Hello, Mrs. Johnson. It's Linda at Dr. Wilson's office. This is your courtesy call to let you know we're looking forward to seeing you tomorrow at 11:00. When you get my message, please call the office's automated voice mail, even if it's after hours, so I'll know you received this important call." Notice the message doesn't say, "...to tell us whether you'll keep the appointment" but rather "please assure me that you received my message."

All these scheduling strategies send a powerful message about what it means to do business with your dental practice: "Rest assured that we treat our patients with the same seriousness and attention to detail that we treat our scheduling policies."

Now that's a message that would put any patient at ease...and coming back for years.

CHAPTER 6

Emergency Patients Are Great Practice Builders

SINCE AN EMERGENCY IS ANY PATIENT WHO NEEDS IMMEDIATE attention, emergencies are what I call an "instant priority." And it's for this very reason, the demand for immediate attention and action, that many offices shy away from emergencies, viewing them as costly interruptions of their day. Nothing could be further from the truth!

Patients in pain or in need of an appointment quickly become every practice's best missionaries. They will tell multiple people if they were treated with dignity and respect. They will tell even more people if their cry for help was treated with total disregard or not at all. Turning away those in pain in fact is anti-marketing one's own practice.

During an after-dinner lecture one evening, I talked about the monetary value of an emergency patient. One dentist interrupted to say, "I hate to dispute what you're saying, but emergency patients in my office aren't worth very much. In fact, they don't even pay their $65 extraction fee." Later that same evening, another doctor came up to see me and said, "Linda, don't ever stop preaching how important emergency patients are. Just a month ago, I had an opportunity to see two of that doctor's patients. One case is over $4,000 and the other is about $2,000. If he doesn't send another patient for six years, we are still ahead of your statistics."

Dental practices who make it a policy not to welcome emergencies could be missing $80,000 and even as much as $200,000 a year in dentistry...and even more in goodwill. If you take good care of emergency patients, they will return to their homes and offices and tell everyone how great they were treated when they needed it most. In fact, emergency patients who are well treated can often be counted on for $1,000 per year in continued care and referrals. On another level, helping people in need gives everyone on the staff a good feeling about themselves, the practice, and the dental profession.

With so much to gain, some offices—perhaps even yours—must change their attitudes about emergencies—and their scheduling strategies to match.

Emergency Flex Time

A well equipped and staffed office can handle two or three emergencies per day without disrupting the schedule. Emergency patients can be examined, x-rayed, anesthetized, and then returned to the reception room while the scheduled patients are seen on time. After the emergency patient's immediate discomfort has been relieved with an anesthetic, he or she should be content to wait until they can be worked into the schedule. Many offices get the emergency patient in the chair and do not know when to stop treatment. This is an unacceptable practice if scheduled patients are being kept waiting.

Somewhere along the line, for reasons I haven't yet determined, dentists got the message that the best three hours of the day to bring in emergencies are the hour before lunch and the last two hours of the afternoon. Since emergencies are a fact of life in a dental practice, a better strategy is to schedule what I call "Emergency Flex Time."

The hour before lunch and the last two hours of the afternoon should be off limits for emergencies because bringing emergencies in at that time will result in missed lunches and overtime hours at the end of the day. When staff give up their lunch or are forced to work past quitting time, morale goes down and production goes with it. The staff will learn quickly to dislike emergency patients because accepting them interferes with their lunch hour and going home time.

Rather than before lunch or late in the afternoon, schedule emergency flex time mid-morning and mid-afternoon (unless the emergency is a trauma case which would be seen twenty-four hours per day). The amount of that emergency flex time will depend on your individual practice. Some of my clients leave twenty to thirty minutes mid-morning and mid-afternoon, while others leave a full hour mid-morning and mid-afternoon because they have more patients and therefore more emergencies.

Seven Steps

There are seven stages of treating the emergency patient that each practice must be aware of in order to use emergencies as the powerful practice building opportunities they are.

Stage 1: It's essential to demonstrate an attitude of gratitude. Very simply, this means a tone of voice, choice of words, and set of actions that let the emergency patient know the dentist and the rest of the team are there for him. The patient senses that everyone will take good care of him, and find a way to work out financial arrangements that enable him to have the quality of dentistry he deserves. Patients will know that the practice treats every emergency with empathy, concern, dignity, and respect and that everyone in the office is happy to help.

Stage 2: The second stage of the emergency protocol is the training of the business and clinical staff in dealing with emergency "interruptions," which in dynamic dentistry we call "opportunities."

For example, upon learning of an emergency, the office's scheduling coordinator should ask, "How soon can you be here?" The message is clear and soothing—music to the ears of a patient in pain. The office is willing to drop everything to attend to him and his needs. If it's a true emergency, the patient will be in as soon as possible. If the patient says he can't make it in until after work, you can safely assume that this is not an actual emergency and the patient can wait for a regular appointment. This is a tried and true method of differentiating the true emergencies from those of less urgency.

Again, the best time to leave emergency flex time is mid-morning and mid-afternoon, column two, with assistant number two. If an emergency patient does not call, the scheduling coordinator can fill the emergency flex time with someone from the Special Call List (see page 121 for more).

Stage 3: When the emergency patient calls the office, he or she is usually in distress; therefore, the scheduling coordinator's tone of voice must be caring, empathetic, and kind.

Getting important needed information from the patient to aid the dentist in his or her diagnosis is also very important during this initial conversation. Answers to questions like, "How long has the tooth been bothering you?" and "Is it sensitive to hot or cold?" often help the dentist determine the nature and severity of the emergency.

Emergency patients should never leave the initial phone call without the emergency fee being presented, simply but clearly: "Mrs. Baxter, I need to let you know that all emergency visits are due and payable at the time of treatment. For your convenience, in addition to cash and personal checks, we also accept Visa and MasterCard."

Stage 4: During the treatment of each emergency, the patient should be aware of the fact that the dentist and entire staff have empathy for their problem. They should never feel rushed or a burden on the practice. They should know, however, that they're being accommodated into a busy schedule, so the appointment may consist of alleviating the pain and then rescheduling the balance of the treatment. Even when this is the case, the office's "We're here to help you" attitude must shine through.

Stage 5: Many start-up practices that are in dire need of more patients overwhelm the emergency patient to return for additional treatment. They say things like, "Mr. Phillips, in treating the emergency situation today, I see many other dental problems that need to be cared for. We'll need to get you back for a complete mouth exam, necessary x-rays, etc. etc. etc."

Often just out of embarrassment, the emergency patient commits to the next appointment but has no intention of returning. These types of emergency patients are truly only interested in "break and fix" care. They also give all emergency patients a bad reputation by not showing up for the next appointment.

I did a mini survey recently that revealed that on average eight out of ten no-shows were patients who were emergencies whom the dentist talked into coming back for a complete oral health exam.

Rather than using this overzealous—and ineffective—approach to reappointing, it's better for the doctor to say, "Mr. Phillips, in doing your emergency examination, I see other dental problems that are about to happen. Here is my business card with our telephone number. When you get tired of having dental pain and dental emergencies, please give Donna, my scheduling coordinator, a call so that she can reserve an hour appointment to do a complete mouth examination and your necessary x-rays. Then, you and I can sit down to discuss the extent of these dental problems and how we can correct them."

Most emergency patients who hear this sort of gentle but firm and sensible advice make the appointment while they are there and keep the appointment because they now "own the problem." That is, they understand it and feel in control of it. They don't feel forced into anything but rather totally in control of their dental destiny.

Stage 6: After each emergency patient has been seen, the dentist or a designated staff member should make a follow-up call within twenty-four hours to see how well the patient is doing and to answer any questions. In doing this, the practice establishes the fact they truly care for all patients, not just patients of record. This measure of goodwill is the "bow on the package" that results in a positive image of the dentist and the practice among patients and the community. And it costs just pennies of time as opposed to hundreds or even thousands of sales promotion and marketing dollars.

Stage 7: Letting the staff know at staff meetings and in casual conversations just how important emergency patients really are is invaluable to the practice's continued growth. Saying things such as, "I don't sign your paycheck; our patients do. The better we care for them the better all our paychecks will be" enables the staff to make it their personal mission to go the extra mile to serve emergency patients, and all patients for that matter.

CHAPTER 7

Collections and Insurance in the Dynamic Dental Practice

COLLECTING FEES ON TIME AND WITH CONSISTENCY REQUIRES A positive attitude, solid collection policies that are applied without exception, and excellent communication skills.

Now in a perfect world, the dentist, assistants, and/or hygienist provides care and the patient pays for that care in full while scheduling his next appointment on the way out. In the rare instances in which someone has forgotten his wallet or checkbook, he leaves with a walk-out statement and an envelope pre-addressed to the office with the understanding that the amount is due immediately.

In a perfect world.

Which doesn't exist.

In the real world, there are many sharp curves and even a pothole or two on the road to the bank; this chapter will provide you with a good map and a set of shock absorbers for the journey.

In dynamic dentistry, accounts receivable are at a comfortable level (no higher than one month's production figure, and preferably even lower) as a direct result of good collections policies and consistent follow-up, including regular statements and collection calls on overdue amounts.

Many dynamic dental practices have just one-tenth of their monthly production in accounts receivable. These practices rarely have cash flow problems.

The reality is that most dental practices have high accounts receivable. Fortunately, this is absolutely unnecessary in today's world of dentistry. First, a look at the reasons:

The primary reason dental practices have high accounts receivable is a lack of collections guidelines. So step 1, which I'll review in a moment, is to sit down as a team and create written financial guidelines. Everything should be covered: How will we handle emergencies financially? How will we handle cases that involve large treatment plans. What about lab procedures, and after insurance co-payments? There should be a clear, agreed-upon guideline for every type of dentistry the practice provides.

The second reason dental practices have high accounts receivable is that the doctor does not stand behind the office guidelines. When the doctor says, "This is how we're going to handle this particular financial situation" but proceeds to make exceptions to this guideline on a regular basis, the guideline becomes meaningless. Exceptions become the rule, and the accounts receivable soars.

The third reason is the staff has never been properly trained to speak about financial matters with patients, and therefore they don't feel competent or confident having these conversations, especially when the topic is a past due balance or high fee. The result is that they simply shy away from talking finances; patients follow suit. And in many practices the staff are loyal to the patients' wallets, not the practice's bottom line.

The fourth reason practices have high accounts receivable is that the staff person responsible for handling collections and insurance—the financial coordinator—is too busy to set aside the time to focus on these all-important tasks.

As management consulting has evolved over the past four decades, those of us who analyze the success and growth of dental practices have become increasingly aware that the total health of a practice can be predicted by the quality of its accounts receivable management.

Consider the fact that patients who owe the practice money are the ones who regularly break appointments. In fact, the number one reason patients cancel appointments is that they have an outstanding balance and have some level of discomfort or embarrassment about facing the staff while their balance isn't paid. These patients also rarely refer other patients, and if they do, they tend to have the same bad habits!

Clear up accounts receivable problems, and you clear up many other problems in the process.

A Valuable Service

Your number one priority when it comes to collections is to keep foremost in everyone's mind the fact that the practice is providing a valuable service essential to the health and well being of its patients. Any time you begin to doubt this for any reason, I want you to think about how much the average person spends on a haircut or a health club membership. People don't seem to mind handing over a credit card or writing a check for these sorts of things—expenses that don't begin to compare in importance to dental care.

Never hesitate to charge appropriately for a procedure that is valuable and essential to people's health and well being. And do not indulge in the delusion that the patients in your town don't want or can't afford quality, comprehensive dentistry. On the contrary, patients from all walks of life will want and be happy to pay for good, comprehensive dentistry when the doctor and the staff believe they deserve the very best.

If you're concerned about your fees for any reason, there are a number of ways to check their competitiveness. First, though, you must know that it is illegal for members of a certain profession or industry to collude, that is to get together to compare or set fees—a practice called price fixing. There are, however, fee surveys available to the dental professional through dental journals and companies that provide an annual fee update based on zip codes, and median fee ranges by service for those zip codes. Some dental study clubs have anonymously placed their fees into a basket and had a listing of highs and lows to share with their membership. Obtain and review these figures, making adjustments to your fees if needed.

Note too that Dr. Charles Blair of Blair, McGill, and Hill of Charlotte, North Carolina, conducts a two-hour Telephone Revenue Enhancement Program that evaluates lost revenue due to fees, poor coding of insurance procedures, and the mix of services. They can be reached at www.bmh-group.com.

An Evolution

In the sixties, it was unheard of to ask patients to pay for services at the time they received treatment. "Good doctors" would provide treatment, send statements, and hope that their "good patients" included the dental practice in their payables that month. Patients would pay $10 to $20 dollars per month on balances that were greater than their monthly incomes! Fees weren't presented at the time of treatment; in fact, money was never exchanged in the office, and if the patient asked about the fee, the response was, "We'll send you a bill."

In the seventies we became a bit less intimidated about being paid for the services provided. Dental seminar content included strategies for presenting fees before the patient left the office after an appointment. Unfortunately, during this transition phase, staff charged with presenting fees more often than not timidly held their heads low and murmured, "The charge for today is $__. How would you like to pay?" or even worse, "Would you like to take care of it?" (We now know never to ask in this way, but rather to simply and professionally explain, "Mrs. Jones, your fee for today is $250. Will that be cash, check, or bank card?" because we now know that if we expect payment, we receive payment!)

Through the eighties and nineties and up to the present, dental practices have made significant strides in accounts receivable management. The notion of "pay as you go" and financing arrangements with financial partners have changed the face of accounts receivable completely. Some practices have chosen to be insurance-free, a decision that has merit in my mind for certain practices, but not others. (More on this later in this chapter.)

Each of these developments in turn has helped to remove financial barriers between patients and the dental care they need, enabling patients to undergo extensive treatment plans in affordable ways. As a result, there has been a surge in the numbers of patients accepting treatment plans which of course translates into large increases in both realized and potential production.

Dental Financing Companies

There are about six well-known and reputable dental financing companies as of this writing. If you're familiar with these organizations, you know just how valuable they are for increasing treatment acceptance. If not, a brief explanation: once the patient agrees and completes a short registration form, the dental financing company establishes the patient's credit rating and then deposits the full amount of the fee for the treatment plan into the dentist's bank account, less a percentage (ranging from seven to ten percent) that the financing company retains as its fee. The dentist is said then to have "no recourse," which means that the financing company is responsible for collecting the fee from the patient directly. The patient, for his part, is receiving a twelve month interest-free loan for the treatment costs on much-needed dentistry. The dentist is out of the picture entirely, and the practice saves on the financial coordinator's time and energy that would otherwise be spent collecting accounts receivable.

It is estimated that practices lose between seventeen and twenty-five percent of the fee handling billings in-office, not to mention the loss of time that could be spent on other, more productive, tasks. What a tremendous boon this makes dental financing companies to treatment acceptance, office efficiency, and low accounts receivable! These arrangements are a win for the practice, the patient, and the financing company.

Picture this scenario, based on a true story: a patient insisted that she would not even consider treatment without a predetermination of benefits from her insurance carrier in front of her to review. Her husband happened to be in full treatment at the time. About six weeks after requesting a predetermination, the financial coordinator called the patient to say, "Shirley, I have some great news. In today's mail, we received your predetermination and it looks as if your employee benefits will cover approximately fifty percent of the total treatment, which means your co-payment will be approximately $1,300." The moment the patient heard $1,300, she said, "I think I'll wait until my husband has finished with his treatment. I didn't expect it to be that much."

With a dental financing company such as Care Credit (www.carecredit.com 800-300-3046) in the picture, the financial coordinator was able to say to the patient, "Shirley, I have some great news. In today's mail, we received your predetermination and it looks as if your employee benefits will cover approximately fifty percent of the total treatment. If I can secure for you a twelve-month interest-free loan on the after-insurance portion, this would translate into $108 a month." The patient accepted the treatment plan right away.

Patients receiving long-term treatments such as crown and bridge, implants, surgery, or complete reconstructive care should know in advance what their total investment will be. On these larger treatments, I highly recommend a retainer fee of twenty-five to fifty percent of the total fee for the next appointment if it is two hours or more of the dentist's time. The verbal skill for this would be, "Mr. Johnson, in order to reserve a half day of the doctor's time, $1,000 of the $4,000 total fee is due and payable five days before the appointment. If you would like to take care of that today, I can process your bank card now or take the information now, and process the fee five days prior to the appointment. Which would you prefer?"

Changing Policies

Many dentists are apprehensive about changing their financial policies—afraid of somehow alienating a patient by the change. In truth, there is some reason for this apprehension. People simply don't like policy changes, particularly if a policy favors them and/or has been in place for a long time. What makes the difference between a policy change that frustrates and alienates patients and one that does not?

The two magic ingredients, not surprisingly, are attitude and proactivity.

The change must be handled with confidence, tact, and professionalism, and it must be introduced in a reasonable time frame, never over night.

I've consulted with many dentists who've purchased an existing practice with high accounts receivable and patients for whom specific payment policies have never been enforced. Every guideline is made to be broken, every case an exception. The result: spoiled patients who resist change at every turn. I advise dentists in these situations to talk to all team members to identify the problems, create policies to alleviate them, commit those policies to writing, and then secure the staff's commitment and support in instituting the policies.

Next, the financial coordinator and/or the dentist should draft a letter to each patient of record detailing key policy changes and the ways in which these changes will actually benefit patients. For example—"As our practice has grown, rather than hire another full-time employee to manage our accounts receivable, which would increase our fees twenty to twenty-five percent, we decided to pass that savings along to our patients by changing the way in which we handle those accounts." Here's another example of stating a policy change in a way that focuses on the benefits to the patient: "We've added electronic billing for insurance. This means that effective [date], if you choose to pay your dental fee at the time of service with a bank card, your insurance reimbursement will arrive often in about ten days—possibly before your bank card statement."

The letter should be kept short with the main goal of patient relationship-building. That is, it should explain the ways in which the change benefits the patient. Any detailed information about the impact of the change should be placed in an attachment to the letter. And, most important, the change should become effective no sooner than ninety days from the date of the letter to give patients time to absorb the information. It can be mailed in monthly statements and presented at checkout to those not receiving statements.

The Financial Options Sheet

Clearly, a dynamic dental practice never operates without written financial guidelines the whole staff is familiar with.

The second must-have, is a financial options sheet for practices that are not cash only. The sheet essentially gives the patient the option of choosing to pay in one of several ways.

The patient is asked to simply circle the one he's most comfortable with. Here's a sample you can feel free to copy and use for your practice:

Doctor's Name and Address **FINANCIAL OPTIONS**

Patient's Name____

Address____

City________________________________State____Zip______

Home Phone ______________Work Phone ______________

Cell number______________ e-mail address______________

I choose the following method of payment for dental care performed for myself and my immediate family:

I Have No Dental Insurance

- ❑ I elect to pay by cash___, check___, Master Card___, Visa____, or Discover ____ on all visits as treatment progresses.

- ❑ I prefer to use your in-office finance plan and to make smaller monthly payments over an extended period of time. I realize that on approved credit, I will qualify interest free for 6 to 12 months.

- ❑ On extensive treatment, I elect to pay 25 percent as a retainer when the treatment is scheduled, 50 percent of the total treatment at the appointment time, and the balance of 25 percent on the delivery or cementation date.

I have Dental Insurance
Name of Insurer: ______________________
Type of Plan:__________________________
Plan or Group #:_______________________

- ❑ I elect to pay my deductible and any co-payment on each visit as treatment progresses.

- ❑ On extensive treatment, I elect to pay 25 percent as a retainer when the treatment is scheduled, 50 percent of the total treatment at the appointment time, and the balance of 25 percent on the delivery or cementation date.

- ❑ On extensive treatment, I elect to pay 50 percent of my co-payment on the preparation date and have the balance placed on my Visa ___, MasterCard ___, or American Express Card ___ in three equal monthly payments.

Signed________________ OR ____________________
Patient Responsible Party

The Dentist's Unwavering Support

Now, in order for policies and guidelines to work effectively, everyone, including the dentist, must adhere to them. I mention this as crucial because one of the most prevalent causes of escalating Accounts Receivable is what I call the "Dr. Nice Guy/Gal" syndrome. A patient approaches the dentist and says, "Doctor, I really want to have the treatment we just discussed, but I don't know how I'm going to afford it." Dr. Nice Guy/Gal, in order to be popular with this person, says, "No problem. I'm sure we can work something out," which is the same as saying, "Money is the least of my concerns. In fact, I don't even care if you pay me." This most definitely is the wrong message to send.

As a general rule, the dentist should NOT be involved in billing, collection, or making financial arrangements. Dentists provide treatment and clinical information. Getting them involved in this aspect of the operation confuses patients about the doctor's role. It's hard for the dentist to show deep concern about the patient's needs and a corresponding treatment plan and then discuss fees without seeming to have a conflict of interest. The patient might think, "Is he suggesting this dentistry just so he can make more money?"

In contrast, when a dentist doesn't get involved in this aspect of the business and doesn't even seem to pay attention to it (though of course he or she does, behind the scenes), the patient is more likely to know that the doctor's primary concern is the health of his teeth.

When Dr. Nice Guy/Gal makes exceptions to office policy, it will only backfire as receivables increase and patients begin to eventually resent the financial coordinator's attempts to enforce office policy. The financial coordinator will have to deal with these patients in the future and will be blamed when patients get behind as a result of Dr. Nice Guy/Gal's intervention. In this scenario, the financial coordinator, of course, is the money-hungry stick-in-the-mud, while Dr. Nice Guy/Gal is an easy-going person who doesn't care about money. Not the chemistry you want to establish for your dynamic dentistry practice!

Instead of opting to be Dr. Nice Guy/Gal, the dentist who's been asked by a patient to reduce or forgive payments should respond with, "Betty, my financial coordinator handles all our financial arrangements. I'm certain she can help you." Patients will be comforted by the doctor's confidence and obvious respect for his staff, and this will help to solidify the patient's relationship with the entire office. And since patient relationships are the heart of every dental practice, I'd say that's mission accomplished!

Clinical staff can also help to convey this message that the financial coordinator handles the money issues by saying as they hand the patients their charts at the end of the treatment, "Please give this to Betty at the front desk. She'll be giving you a receipt for today's visit."

Staff Competence and Confidence

For some reason, the subject of money causes many people to squirm in discomfort, avoid eye contact, and drop their voices down to a barely audible whisper, as if earning a living is something to be ashamed of! First of all, it isn't, especially when your office provides a service of value and importance in people's lives and you've got the education and training needed and have made significant investments in technology and equipment in order to deliver this service with superior quality.

Second, this discomfort is the classic self-fulfilling prophecy: you will find that if you behave in a way that suggests you are undeserving of your fees, patients will begin to believe that you are indeed undeserving and they will respond accordingly with late payments, slow responses to your calls about overdue payments, and other forms of resistance and postponement.

On the other hand, when your staff is trained to present your fees clearly, calmly, and in a pleasantly professional manner and without an apology, either explicit or implicit, patients react accordingly: fees are honored payments are made on time, and calls are returned promptly.

> One of dynamic dentistry's "never-use" phrases is "payment arrangement." This is a term from the 1970s that's almost always used to mean a patient will settle a balance due the practice by paying $10 a month for the rest of his life!

Although collection rests in the hands of the practice's financial coordinator, all staff members should feel knowledgeable about the practice fee and able to successfully conduct a fee rebuttal. (See pages 150, 201, and

202 for examples.) The entire staff must be thoroughly proactive in conversations with patients about fees and financial arrangements. No information about these topics should come as a surprise to a patient. My philosophy has always been that to surprise a patient is often to lose a patient.

Presenting Fees

Fees should always be presented at the desk. Upon checkout, the patient should be escorted to the financial coordinator by the clinical staff member who walks the patient to the desk and says, "Mrs. Jones, it was great seeing you today. I look forward to your next visit. I've given your chart to our financial coordinator, Diane. She will be giving you your receipt for today's visit."

If your practice accepts assignment of insurance benefits, the statement might be, "Mrs. Jones, it was great seeing you today. I look forward to your next visit. I've given your chart to our financial coordinator, Diane. She'll be processing your insurance immediately and giving you a receipt for your co-payment.

Listen to the powerful messages implicit in this simple act:

- ✧ We take care of you from the moment you arrive to the moment you leave. I will help you get your bearings and personally escort you to the desk.
- ✧ It was good to see you.
- ✧ I look forward to next time.
- ✧ Diane will take it from here.
- ✧ We expect payment now, and will be happy to issue your receipt right away.

When every hygienist and every dental assistant in a dynamic dental practice gets in the habit of saying this, the practice's over-the-counter collections increase dramatically.

All fees for each day's visit should be presented to the patient as he stands at the desk scheduling the next appointment. In presenting this information, use positive language filled with the highest expectations:

reappoint the patient, then smile and say, "Mrs. Brown, the fee for today's visit is $[amount]. Will you be paying by cash, check, or credit card today?"

Present fees to patients with insurance coverage as usual at the end of a visit following reappointment, but with a bit of a different presentation: "Mr. Jones, the fee for today's visit is $[amount]. We'll be filing your insurance immediately for you as a courtesy. Your approximate portion is $[amount]. Will you be paying that by cash, check, or credit card today?"

Every member of the team in your practice must know how to present fees effectively. This is for two reasons: first, the financial coordinator may be on vacation or temporarily unavailable at a the time fees need to be presented, and second, because everyone with patient contact—and in a dental practice, that IS everyone—will be asked questions from time to time about fees and financial policies. It's essential that patients get the message loud and clear that this is a team with solid policies that speaks in one clear, coherent voice about them.

If a patient's treatment is $1,000, his insurance covers $700, and his portion is $300, say, "Mr. Wilson, your employee benefit plan will be covering approximately $700 of the $1,000 fee. Your portion will be approximately $300. Will that be cash, check, or bank card? Notice I've inserted the word "approximately" and this is very deliberate. When insurance is involved, it's best to be a bit circumspect. Many policies have complexities and special provisions that can increase or decrease the amount of expected payment.

Think of the last purchases you made. Did you expect a fee discount? Did the seller apologize for taking your hard-earned money? Did they ask if you'd like to pay for your groceries or just send a check when you want? Of course not. Your practice will never become "big business" until you run it as such.

A Solid Collection System

> When collections are handled properly, about ninety-five percent of dental patients can be expected to pay on time, about three percent will pay eventually, and about two percent will never pay.

What is your office's collection rate?

1. Total monthly monies collected from patients and insurance companies: ________
2. Total monthly production: ________
3. Subtract any adjustments from production for staff or family members, insurance write-offs, etc.: ____________________
4. Divide collections by the adjusted production: ___________
5. Move the decimal two places to the right: _______________

Any dental practice can have up to a ninety-eight percent annual collection rate through strong collection policies and practices.
Bear in mind that the ninety-eight percent figure is an average. So, if you have a lower than ninety percent collection ratio one month, strive for a more than one hundred percent collection the following month. Also remember that if the accounts receivable balance is excessive, the collection goals should be well over one hundred percent each month until accounts receivable reaches an acceptable level.

Statements

Statements are mailed out only to those patients with true outstanding balances, not those with insurance pending. If your office accepts insurance, never send a statement to a patient for a past due amount that is actually a pending insurance payment because you will cause a great deal of expense and confusion in doing so. The patient will call and say, "Linda I just got this statement from you, and I thought you knew that we had insurance, We talked about it." "Oh, yes, just disregard the statement. We're waiting for the insurance check. It's not overdue yet." Not a great message to send to patients to disregard any correspondence from your office. In addition, this seems to suggest that you're not on top of paperwork, submissions, insurance practices, and the like.

If there's a delay in the insurance check and the patient receives a second statement, another confused call from the patient comes in, a bit more exasperated this time: "Linda, haven't you received my insurance yet? I just got another statement from you!" "Yes, well disregard that one too. We're expecting the payment any day now." By the time the insurance payment arrives, if there's a difference the office has to bill for, guess what the patient is going to do with the statement? That's right: disregard it, just like the other ones.

In solo practices, I recommend mailing statements on the fifteenth of each month with a due date the fifth of the following month. Delinquent calls must be made as soon as the account becomes past due by thirty days. Another strategy in a two-doctor practice is to mail A through M statements on the tenth and N through Z statements on the twentieth to keep the office cash flow even. Bear in mind that some practices today perform billing on a daily basis, with a due date ten days from the date the statement is generated. Imagine never having to do batch billing again or having angry patients because their accounts are just sitting there waiting for a prompt from you! With instant billing daily, patients know you mean business.

If your office accepts insurance, make sure you have a policy that you can only wait a maximum of sixty days for all insurance checks. When the insurance check is not received within thirty days, call the patient and let them know that if the insurance check is not received,within another thirty days they will become financially responsible for the fee. Then give them the insurance company's toll-free number so that the patient may do their own insurance inquiry. After all, you have hundreds of claims and they have only one or two. (Insurance companies act faster when the subscribers contact them than when the dental office does. So, getting the patient involved brings immediate results in most cases.) Call the patient and explain, "Ms. Jones, this is Linda from Dr. Brown's office. We mailed your insurance claim in the amount of $178 on February 12. I'm calling since it's now the middle of March, and the insurance check has not been received. We can wait a maximum of sixty days for all insurance checks. By the twelveth of next month, if the insurance check has not been received, we'll ask that you pay the $178. If and when the insurance company sends a check, we will be happy to reimburse you."

Dentists should ask for a computer-generated insurance report monthly. Study it to see how many claims have not been paid and why. Total the amount and have someone go to work on these assured accounts receivable immediately. The outstanding amounts can be earth shattering in some practices.

Collecting Past-Due Accounts

Before making collection calls, the dentist and staff must be aware of state and federal laws governing collections. These laws apply to everyone making these calls, including a collection agency hired by the dentist. If the agency does not abide by these laws, the dentist can be held liable. So awareness is essential.

You can get a copy of these laws by contacting your local credit bureaus, the Retail Merchants Association nearest you, or on the Internet under state and federal agencies.

A phone call is proven to be much more effective than a collection letter. The caller must be well versed in collection tactics to be effective. These calls are designed to make both the staff member and patient feel comfortable while collecting amounts due. With this in mind, the caller must:

- ✧ Never lose control.
- ✧ Be courteous and calm.
- ✧ Speak clearly.
- ✧ Establish a definite financial arrangement before ending the conversation by securing two verbal agreements during the conversation: the date the payment will be received, and the amount of the payment.
- ✧ Create a written and computerized record of the promised amount and date.
- ✧ Never argue about money.
- ✧ Keep a positive attitude. It is important to feel you are performing a valuable service for the office. If you do not feel comfortable making collection calls, you must learn to overcome this and master this skill. It's that essential.

Collection calls must be made monthly for all overdue accounts. The first past-due call should be made within days after the payment due date. Calls should be made at a time when the collections person is in a position to devote uninterrupted time to the task. Remember that you may only speak directly to the person responsible for making the payment or that person's spouse on joint accounts.

Kindness and empathy are essential to collections success. When making collection calls over the years, I actually became friendly with patients I called each month. If patients have temporary financial problems, it is always the "nice" collectors who get paid first when their finances improve.

Be firm, polite, and to the point. "Hello, Mrs. Webber. This is Joan from Dr. Wood's office. I am calling in regard to your outstanding balance of $150. We haven't received a payment since March 3. There must be a problem." In stating that "there must be a problem," you're giving the patient an opportunity to offer an explanation in a non-defensive manner.

Be sympathetic to the explanation the patient provides, then continue with: "I'm so sorry to hear that, but our accountant was in last week to review our accounts. He'll be back next week for a report on this overdue account. May I please tell him what day of each month you will send a payment and what the amount that payment will be?"

I've found that using an outside "ghost" of an accountant removes the "bad guy" image from the office and makes the conversation more comfortable for the patient and staff person. And, as Zig Ziglar says, "You shouldn't tell a lie, but you can tell the truth in advance." If your accounts receivable increase, your accountant will ask why!

Let's build this scenario a bit further. Suppose the patient's response is, "My husband handles all our finances, so I cannot give you the date or an amount." You reply, "That's fine, Mrs. Webber. Please discuss it with him tonight and I'll call back tomorrow for your answer." And, always follow through.

When you finally reach Mrs. Webber the next day, she commits to sending $40 on the 15th of each month. Enter this in the computer notes of the patient's account.

If the patient becomes threatening or argumentative, calmly end the conversation with, "I obviously caught you at a bad time. I'll call again."

A second collection call is necessary whether or not the patient has paid as promised.

If the patient has paid, you call to say, "Hello, Mr. Wells. This is Alice from Dr. Rolen's office. I'm calling to thank you for your $50 payment, which we received on January 12. We'll expect the same amount by the 12th of next month and appreciate your cooperation in clearing the account."

If the patient hasn't paid, continue to call using the language used in the initial call until the balance is paid. Persistence is key; experience shows that when the calls stop, often the payments do as well.

Set up a 1 to 31 tickler system in the computer to check daily for amounts that were promised but not paid, and follow up accordingly. For example, on the eighteenth of the month, check back three numbers to day fifteen. If the $40 payment promised on that date beside the patient's name has not arrived, the patient should receive a second call that month. "Mr. White, this is Jenny from Dr. Nolen's office. The payment of $40 you promised on the fifteenth has not been received, and today is the eighteenth. If it is not in the mail already, I would appreciate it if you would bring it by the office or place it in today's mail."

A few patients give repeated, unkept promises that waste time and create stress for the financial coordinator. After several attempts produce only empty promises, send the patient a final notice. This can be a form notice or a letter from an attorney or a collection agency.

I don't usually recommend using a collection agency because they keep a large percentage of what they collect, and attorneys usually only handle large accounts. The good news is that if the office systematically keeps its accounts under control, outside services are not necessary.

Credit Cards

Clearly display the Visa, MasterCard, and American Express logos and the logos of any other cards the office accepts, and mention credit cards throughout your financial option conversations and as you present fees. Though of course the credit card company keeps a small portion of the payment as its fee, credit cards make collection simple and quick because patient payments are deposited directly into the bank within a day or so. Since they save time and paperwork, credit cards save money too.

If your office is on a cash basis, you might suggest that patients with insurance use a credit card to pay their fee as you instantaneously submit the claim to their insurance carrier. This way, the payment may arrive in time for the patient to use it to pay off the credit card bill, without incurring any interest.

A Solid Framework

So, now you have a solid framework on which to build your dynamic accounts receivable guidelines and practices. To recap, in the dynamic dental practice:

✧ Financial policies and guidelines are clearly written and understood by each member of the team.

✧ The dentist fully supports the guidelines and allows the staff to enforce the policies in the same friendly manner in which the practice delivers the dentistry. The dentist never gets involved or sides with patients who may question the policies. He or she always refers those issues to the practice's financial coordinator.

✧ Staff members are all fully trained with verbal skills in financial discussions. They truly believe in the quality of the dentistry the office delivers and believe the fees are valid and fair. They enjoy defending the fees in a positive manner when patients question the fees. The practice has invested in a creative financing plan to make it easy for the staff to collect fees in a positive, non-threatening manner. The dentist's attitude toward this plan is highly positive.

✧ The dentist allows the financial coordinator to reserve one to four hours weekly to work on twenty-five percent of the alphabet on any past dues patients or insurance accounts. This person is fully trained to make professional and effective collection calls. The financial coordinator also has the tools to teach patients how to do their own insurance inquiry if there is a non-payment from their benefit plan. Alternatively, the dentist has stood behind the new policy of being insurance-free.

Insurance: Yes or No?

When it comes to a dental practice's approach to insurance, the first rule of thumb is that one size doesn't fit all. Each practice must choose among essentially four options for handling insurance based on their unique needs. These options are:

- ✧ accept assignment on every plan available
- ✧ accept assignment on two or three plans, chosen for their prevalence among patients in your practice
- ✧ accept only indemnity plans—no PPOs or HMOs—with patients paying all co-payments at time of service.
- ✧ go insurance-free (also called a cash practice)

In recent years, there has been a bit of a trend toward creating a cash practice, that is, not accepting insurance as payment for any patients covered under any plan. I advise clients to be extremely careful about making this choice. In some cases, it's appropriate, as in the case of an established practice with more patients than the staff can handle. But for new dentists just beginning to establish a practice, it may be unwise to in effect exclude insurance patients from the practice by not accepting assignment. These dentists should consider Option 2, that is, accept a few plans that are most prevalent among potential patients in the community. (Option 1, accept all plans, is a tough road to travel because of the burden of paperwork and because insurance fees tend to be at a low level.) For new practices, indemnity insurance is another way to quickly and effectively collect accounts receivable and to help build the practice in the process.

For dentists accepting a few carefully selected plans, submit treatment plans for an explanation of benefits before treatment is delivered. If the benefit level is lower than your fees and patients question this, you might want to say simply that your fees are above average because the quality of care you deliver is above average and simply leave it at that. Don't get into a lengthy back and forth about insurance companies and their methods! This conversation is likely to be defensive and even potentially hostile. Simply take the high road and say you made a decision early on not to compromise the quality of care you deliver based on insurance rates or any other factor. Patients need to be aware that the care, skill, and training that enables the practice to deliver superior dental care may cost more than the insurance company's usual and customary fee.

Fee Rebuttal:

"We're extremely proud of our fees—they reflect the quality of care our practice delivers." (See pages 201-202 for additional fee rebuttals)

CHAPTER 8

Preventive Care and Your Recare System: The Best Practice-Building Strategy

THE HYGIENE DEPARTMENT AND PREVENTIVE CARE ARE THE HEART of every successful dental practice. Indeed, these are two of the most powerful practice-building elements of a dynamic dental practice. The reasons are obvious: preventive care is a unique mechanism for maintaining a patient's ongoing relationship with your dental practice, not to mention providing optimum care for each patient. The more often you see patients, the stronger their ties to the practice. This translates into ongoing business and increasing numbers of referrals, making it among the best marketing and practice-building strategies available.

In a dynamic dental practice, the hygiene department generates a third or more of the practice's total volume. If the practice is generating $60,000 for instance, the hygiene department should bring in at least $20,000. (Practices perform this calculation differently. Some dentists count only prophys and initial perio therapy as hygiene production, while others take out the exam because they consider it doctor production. Still others include x-rays, sealants, and whitening trays. If your office counts everything including the doctor exam, hygiene could be as much as forty percent of total volume. If your calculation excludes a number of items, hygiene could comprise as little as twenty-five percent of total volume.

Why is recare in hygiene a practice building system? Because the patients you're not presently seeing in hygiene are the patients who need the most operative, restorative, and cosmetic care.

One more valuable statistic: your recare system fuels the restorative practice and in fact should be responsible for forty to forty-five percent of the restorative practice. Clearly, a large percentage of restorative and cosmetic dentistry comes from the hygiene department.

In my experience consulting with well over 1,100 dental practices, I've seen improvements in hygiene scheduling that start with a long, hard look at a practice's recare system produce the single most phenomenal jumps in production. As hygiene goes, so goes the whole practice…for better or worse!

I've often said that we need to be certain to tell patients who balk at the time and money involved in preventive care that it's not preventive dentistry that's expensive, but rather neglect. The interesting addendum is this: lack of preventive care is not only expensive for the patient…clearly it's expensive for the practice as well.

How Effective Is Your Hygiene Department?

1. Count your active patients (those who have been seen in the past 18-24 months). Example: 2,500
2. Multiply by 2 (as most patients are seen twice per year—some less, some more). Example: 2,500 x 2 = 5000
3. Divide by 12. Example: 5000 / 12 months = approximately 416 recares monthly

The numbers above indicate a need to see 416 patients per month in hygiene. If a practice has only one hygienist who is seeing an average of 7 patients per day, at 16 working days per month, that's 112 patients per month.

Divide 112 patients the hygienist is seeing by the 416 she should be seeing, and it's clear that this hygiene department is only 27 percent effective!

Preventive care and the patient education that goes along with it are also essential to patients' dental health—which makes them a professional responsibility.

I also guarantee that if your office does not effectively recare patients, rest assured that another office will.

Given all this, it's essential that your recare system function like a well-oiled machine, with all bases covered (few patients slipping through the cracks!) and regular, ongoing reappointments and confirmation calls.

Resist the temptation to panic when practice growth slows and to cut expenses by reducing the number of hygiene days. Your first step is to reevaluate the effectiveness of your recare system and take action fast. This is one of the simplest, fastest ways to jumpstart practice growth.

For the new dentists reading this book, please know that not hiring a hygienist within six months of starting a new practice (part-time) is the surest way to slow the growth of your practice. Many non-busy new dentists say, "Why should I hire someone to do preventive care when I'm not that busy?" Sounds logical, but as long as the dentist is spending twenty-five to thirty percent of their day being a hygienist, they are missing an opportunity to do treatment plans the hygienist supports.

My advice to new dentists is to condense your patients into fewer days or hours per week, have a hygienist to do all preventive care, and use the other day or two per week to get out into the community and shake hands with potential patients. Networking or giving community talks is a sure way to become known! (For much more on marketing, see Chapter 10.)

If a new dentist purchases an existing practice, they often think they're saving on overhead by getting rid of the highest paid person on the team. This is truly "stepping over dollars to pick up dimes!" The hygienist and other staff are the bridge to patients' acceptance and trust of the new dentist in most cases.

Dynamic dental practices use hygiene as a practice catalyst and distinguish themselves by doing all they can to work their recare system to the hilt and sharpen it over time.

Three Approaches

There are basically three types of recare systems in dentistry today used by practices striving to meet these goals. First among these—this is not the most prevalent—is the reminder mailing, most often a simple postcard that says some variation of "It's time to call us."

This is the approach I recommend taking if for some reason you're aiming to undermine the effectiveness of your front desk staff or to make them crazy. While this approach gives the patient full responsibility for making their appointments and saves a minute or two during check out, it comes with significant disadvantages. Only twenty to thirty percent of patients call to schedule appointments upon receipt of their recare reminder cards. Patients try to postpone recare intervals. Incoming calls create interruptions. And finally, this system actually results in many emergency appointments due to postponed preventive care for the patient.

The second recare system in use in dentistry—also ineffective—consists of using a Preventive Care Coordinator who spends forty hours a week trying to lasso people back to the hygiene department. This approach adds the expense of another employee in the job with the greatest likelihood of resulting in burnout in a dental practice. I call this the "Call and Recall" approach and it has no known advantages. Calling, calling, and recalling takes hours of staff time and becomes irritating for the patients. It also makes the practice appear desperate for patients and in decline…not the sort of dental practice that inspires patient confidence!

The third and absolute best recare system in dentistry hearkens back to the golden rule of thumb I introduced earlier: no patient ever leaves the office without their next appointment. This is the most powerful patient retention strategy available to you, with numerous advantages: It saves hundreds of hours annually in calling and recalling. When it's done right, there are fewer changed appointments. Since I strongly recommend the hygienist do all the preappointing chairside (more on this starting on page 158), the hygienist has control over her schedule; therefore, difficult patients are not scheduled back to back and patients are scheduled for the exact amount of time they need. The approach is much more professional and less likely to annoy patients than continuous calling. Its only disadvantage is that the dentist and hygienist must select vacation dates three to six months in advance (a small price to pay for doubling retention rates of patients and many hours of tedious calling). And they must leave flexible time in the hygiene schedule (one day a month for continuing education, snow days, or illness). If the hygienist must have a day off for one of these reasons, patients can be moved to the flexible date.

This recare system has added thousands of dollars to the productivity of many offices, and it's saved hours of time for the staff who no longer have to chase recare lists.

Two Must-Haves

There are two must-haves for preappointing to work with maximum effectiveness. First, you cannot wait until the day before a patient's appointment to make your courtesy call on an appointment scheduled three or six months prior. Instead, send a positively worded preconfirmation postcard two weeks before the scheduled appointment and make a courtesy call one or two days prior.

The second must-have if you're going to preappoint is sufficient flex time in your hygiene schedule. You need monthly as well as daily flex time. Using up all your hygiene appointments months in advance would cripple this all-important schedule. Instead, have at least one full day of flex time in each hygienist's schedule each month—that's twelve flex days a year—that you do not start to fill until three weeks in advance of a given day.

On daily flex time, I recommend one to two openings per day (depending on the number of patients in your practice and the number of initial perio patients). Busy practices may need two openings a day in hygiene that aren't scheduled until seventy-two hours in advance. Into these openings go new patient prophys and initial perio patients. How terrible for my hygienist to tell me I have a beginning to moderate degree of periodontal disease in my mouth but she can't see me for several months to begin treatment. This happens in too many practices. By running the monthly production report to see how many perio procedures were done, in practices with no flex time we see four or five initial perio treatments monthly. In offices that leave daily flex time we see four to five times that number.

Once Again, Attitude Matters

The classic objection many people have to my rule about making sure a patient doesn't leave without scheduling his next appointment is that patients either won't like or won't be willing to schedule appointments so far in advance.

Again, though, we find the importance of staff attitude. If the staff doesn't believe in this policy, they'll hesitate, forget, put it off with one patient, and then with another and another. Before long, preappointing will no longer be standard practice.

On the other hand, as is the case with any office policy that affects patients, if the staff accepts the approach and sees it as the best means for solidifying patient relationships and presents it to patients accordingly, patients will respond positively. Once again, the attitude and verbal skills of the staff and doctors determines the success of any policy, especially one that involves a change.

> A patient with an appointment for three, six, nine, or twelve months is a committed patient—your patient!

Here are some proven-effective strategies for handling this essential communication with patients:

- ✧ Rather than phrase reappointment as a question ("Linda we need to see you again in four months. Do you want to go ahead and make that appointment while you're here?"), make a statement: "If this time is good for you, Linda, let's reserve the same time in four months."

- ✧ If a patient says she'd rather have you call in four months to schedule the next appointment—an inevitability roughly ten percent of the time—respond by explaining, "If you reserve the appointment now, you'll have your choice of time and day. If you wait, you're likely to have fewer choices of appointment dates and times."

- ✧ If a patient says he'll never remember an appointment scheduled so far in advance, assure him with a statement like: "Of course, we will confirm your appointment with a card two weeks in advance and a courtesy call the day before." (Order the Linda Miles Signature recare cards from www.hycomb.com)

- ✧ If the patient asks whether any other patients want to schedule appointments far in advance, answer in the affirmative and help them to know they're in good company: "We find that patients find it easier to schedule in advance because nothing is competing for their time, and they can plan around this important appointment."

- ✧ If the patient explains he doesn't have the money to come on a regular basis, remind him that preventive care is far less costly than emergency care by saying, "Mr. Patient, maintaining your teeth is much like maintaining your car. A maintenance visit is far less costly than a new transmission or engine" or "Dr. Johnson likes to find small dental problems before they develop into major dental emergencies" or "I'm sure you'll agree that coming for preventive care regularly is well worth the investment of time and money when you think of the alternatives."

- ✧ Treat the reappointment as an important health-related event rather than just a check-up. In many practices I hear conversations such as: "Let's go ahead and book your next CLEANING or CHECK-UP." These words make the appointment sound insignificant and unimportant, encouraging cancellation or no-shows. Use instead, "preventive care appointment," "continuous care appointment." or "follow-up care appointment."

- ✧ The practice of preappointing hygiene sends several important and positive message to your patients:
    - "We are so efficient that we plan this far ahead of the game."

- "We need to plan because we're so in demand."
- "Your preventive care appointments are so important to us that we reserve the time exclusively for you months in advance."
- "Our emphasis on hygiene is intended to save you time, money, and discomfort down the line."

Establishing a Chairside Preappointing System

Preappointing patients for hygiene recare appointments the day the patient is in the office is a great practice-building and patient retention strategy, but to enable it to reach its full potential, the hygienist (or the hygiene assistant in an assisted hygiene model) must conduct all the preappointing chairside. (In making this recommendation, I'm counting on the fact that in today's world of dentistry, you have a terminal in each hygiene room.)

There are several reasons why your hygienist should make his or her own appointments chairside. First, having the hygienist preappoint at this time takes one minute per patient but can save the office about twenty hours a month of time because it saves a dozen reappointments each day for the scheduling coordinator. Patients are far more receptive to scheduling their next appointment in a clinical setting with the hygienist than in a busy business office with its many distractions.

Next, not all hygiene patients require the same amount of time. The hygienist knows this better than anyone in the office and can develop the schedule accordingly.

This has the effect of instantly improving the quality of the relationship between your hygienist and your business staff because with the hygienist in complete control of her schedule, she'll never have a reason to blame the front desk staff for putting two difficult patients back to back, preventing her from leaving on time, or any other scheduling problem.

Since patients are preappointed chairside as part of the patient education process, there is less of a bottleneck at the front desk. Patients come out, pay, and leave. In the not-too-distant future, "Quick Pay" chairside will evolve, which means the credit card swipe will be done in the treatment room allowing the hygiene patient to pay, be treated and not have to stop at the desk. This is the continuation of the early '80s "frontdesklessness" idea (see page 84). Again, a concept that is good in theory but not in practice. In my opinion, as good as it may seem, a greeter is still appreciated by the patients and necessary to have the phones handled promptly. Terminals chairside have been a plus, but what I believe will evolve in this wonderful profession of dentistry is a kind of Dental Concierge! No form of automation could replace the civility and warmth of a personal greeting.

There are also fewer broken appointments in hygiene because the commitment is between the patient and the hygienist.

Here are some guidelines to help you implement a chairside preappointing system in hygiene:

1. Each hygienist must have a computer terminal chairside. Alternatively, there must be a hygiene department computer in the hallway used by all hygienists.

2. With computerized scheduling, the computer generates the continuous feed recare postcard two weeks prior to the appointment. These are efficient but with non-computerized recare cards the patients can pre-address to themselves.

3. If the patient chooses not to make the appointment, the hygienist immediately enters the patient's name, due date, phone number, and units of appointment time into the computer tickler file under the month due.

4. The tickler file is a way to prevent the practice from forgetting patients and their needed treatment, as well as a means of creating a backup list of patients you may wish to call to fill openings in the schedule.

Follow these guidelines for creating a pending appointment system:

No patient leaves the office without either an appointment or their name entered into the computerized pending tickler system.

If a patient cancels an appointment, their name is not deleted until their name has been entered into the Pending Tickler System.

5. The scheduling coordinator mails the pre-confirmation hygiene cards two weeks prior to each patient's appointment.

6. The scheduling coordinator makes courtesy calls to scheduled hygiene appointments. If the hygienist has "down time" she may also make courtesy calls or telemarket lost patients to keep the hygiene schedule filled.

Power Up Your Hygiene Department

I've seen too many practices hesitate to bring in more hygiene business for fear of overwhelming the dentist with patient exams. Perhaps they only have one hygiene room and are concerned about overburdening the hygiene schedule. Step one for these practices—which lose about 250 hygiene patients a month due to this limitation—is to add a second hygiene room, but before hiring an additional hygienist, try getting more hygiene appointments simply by being more effective in your daily scheduling.

Here's one approach I've seen work with tremendous effectiveness. Start by taking four days of operative, restorative, and cosmetic dentistry and condensing them into three days with more effective scheduling and staff utilization (see Chapter 4 for strategies). You've now freed up one additional day a week of your chairside assistants' time and can instantly increase the practice's production in hygiene by having one of the two assistants assist the hygienist.

The production boost this produces is one of the reasons assisted hygiene has become so popular in recent years. Unassisted, a hygienist with one hygiene chair can handle eight to ten patients a day. With a hygiene assistant and two chairs, this number increases to thirteen to fifteen a day. (For much more on assisted hygiene, refer to pages 106-108.)

An alternative to assisted hygiene as a tool to catch up on preventive care patients is "Super Hygiene Day." When there aren't enough treatment rooms to add a hygienist or when the dentist prefers the pace of examining only one hygiene schedule throughout his or her busy day, this strategy could be beneficial.

"Super Hygiene Day" was implemented in several client offices with tremendous success. If an office is losing 200 hygiene patients per month, I recommend condensing the dentist's operative from five to four days or 4.5 to 3.5 days per week and have one day of four chairs (the typical solo practice set up) for assisted hygiene in all four rooms. This is two hygienists and two assistants. The dentist does nothing but patient examinations all day. They now have fewer interruptions plus more time to reinforce the patient's needed dentistry. With each assisted hygiene team seeing fifteen patients each, thirty patients a day multiplied by four days a month provides the dentist with the same number of patients as one full-time hygienist with less stress.

Now, how does the dentist compress a schedule of operative patients from four days to three? The answer is better delegation to well-trained assistants, allowing them to do most of the pre-treatment explanations and post-treatment patient education (see pages 45-46).

While I never advocate sacrificing quality for quantity, please know you can have both. Dental assistants have an entirely new role in the dynamic dental practice. While no one can diagnose or provide a treatment plan except the dentist, the verbally skilled staff can save the dentist seven out of ten minutes per patient by sharing this important task. Interactive patient education tools such as CAESY are also very useful. This technology can be accessed at www.caesy.com.

Wealth of Opportunity

A healthy, active recare system will make any practice busier than ever with nonstop increases in production. For this reason, I consider inactive patients to be the sleeping giant in every dental practice, by which I mean that there is literally a goldmine in most dental office filing systems comprised of files of once active patients. These are those individuals who have not been to see the dentist or hygienist for a year or more.

Once they're contacted, large percentages of these patients rekindle their relationship with the practice translating into thousands of dollars to the bottom line. Why? In my experience because these patients have a degree of familiarity and comfort in the practice. For this reason, it's a great deal easier and less expensive marketing-wise to reconnect with a former patient who knows the practice than it is to start a new relationship altogether, making this a key motivation behind investing the time and energy needed to reach out to these patients.

Dynamic dental practices know how to wake this sleeping giant by systematically reaching out to these patients on a regular basis. To return inactive patients back to the practice as active patients, you might try contacting them by mail. However, this generally produces only a fifteen to twenty-five percent response rate and creates expenses like printing and postage.

A telephone-based process results in a much higher percentage of reappointed patients—up to fifty percent depending upon the communication skills of the caller and the type of patients in the practice (committed versus non-committed). This process of telemarketing inactive patients should be done on an ongoing basis, not haphazardly or just once or twice a year.

If your practice is located in a stable area, with people not moving in and out like in a military town for instance, four to six out of ten patients who are contacted should schedule if the call is handled deftly. Here's a script that works very well:

"Good morning, Mr. Johnson. This is Linda from Dr. Wilson's office. We are updating our patient records for the current year. Your last appointment with our hygienist and Dr. Wilson was fourteen months ago. Because your follow-up care is so important, I'm calling today to reserve a time for you, before all of our hygiene appointments are filled for the next three months."

This positive approach makes many patients realize that the office is calling for their benefit.

A few important notes on word choice:

- ✧ The word "reserve" lends an air of importance to the appointment.
- ✧ Do not say "cleaning" or "check-up or recall." Instead refer to "your last preventive care appointment," "your continuous care," or "your follow-up care."
- ✧ Always look at the date of the patient's last appointment and determine how many months it's been, because the number of

months is more significant than the calendar date. When you mention a date, it doesn't register how long it's been since the patient's last appointment, which is a key part of the message you want to convey.

The best hours to do telemarketing are 9:00 to 11:00 a.m. on Saturday morning, and 4:00 to 6:00 p.m. on weekdays. This is the best time to catch moms at home who are for the most part the decision makers and family scheduling coordinators!

If the patient makes an appointment during the telemarketing campaign, don't forget to invite other family members by saying, "Mrs. Johnson, now that we have you scheduled, how about your other family members who may also be past due for their preventive care appointments?" It's amazing how many times you will get one or more new patients out of this campaign! The key is to ask. It simply doesn't hurt to ask the patient whether your practice can help anyone else, and it's also a sound, cost-effective marketing strategy. You're already on the phone with the patient; by asking for more business, you're maximizing the investment you've already made in patient retention and practice growth.

If a patient has been contacted repeatedly and still has not scheduled, eventually say,"Would you like to make an appointment at this time or be placed in our inactive files?"

Although this may sound like a bit of a harsh ultimatum, it encourages patients to reschedule. No patient wants to be considered "inactive" since this sounds as if the doctor will be unavailable to treat them in an emergency or they may be handled differently if they do choose to return at some point.

If the patient intends to return and has been postponing the next recare appointment, the ultimatum brings the appointment decision to the surface and motivates a response.

There will be times when a patient says, "Go ahead and place me in your inactive files," which usually means the patient is seeing another dentist. Simply say, "Oh, Mr. Johnson, we're sorry we won't be seeing you and your family on a regular basis. Please keep in mind that a call from you is all we need to have you back in our active files." This clearly tells the patient that he or she would be welcomed back to your practice at any point.

Some patients leave for one reason or another often thinking, "The grass may be greener in another practice." Sometimes they realize that it was artificial turf. Having "the door is always open" as a policy and an attitude that permeates the practice enables patients to gracefully return.

Before you close the conversation with a departing or departed patient, always remember to say, "Mr. Johnson, we're sorry we won't be seeing you (and your family) on a regular basis. To complete your record, may I please chart the reason you wish to be inactive?" Remember to record this on their chart or in the computer notes and keep a list of reasons for discussing with the doctor and at your next staff meeting. If you don't know WHY the practice has lost or is losing patients, you will continue to lose them for the same reasons.

Clearly, though it's sometimes not easy to hear, negative feedback from patients is essential to practice growth and longevity. The reactivation call provides an excellent opportunity to extract reasons for dissatisfaction among patients. Simply say, "To complete our records, may I please chart the reason you wish to be inactive?" The patient will almost always give the staff member the true reason, an uncaring attitude on the part of doctors and staff or being kept waiting too long, for instance.

Other reasons patients leave include: 1) "I was never pleased with the shade of my crown," 2) "My treatment plan was not fully discussed before treatment," and 3) "My child's problems didn't seem important to anyone there." In these instances, offer the patient a complimentary consultation appointment to discuss the problem. Many of these hidden problems are rectified easily, and the patients become good missionaries because the practice has demonstrated an obvious desire to satisfy patients. The staff has shown that patients are at the center of all they do.

Identifying Inactive Patients to Contact

Here's a valuable technique for systematically identifying patients to contact for those practices that are not paperless and chartless. To use my technique, you must first be certain you're using year stickers on patient charts for visual as well as computer-generated reports.

- ✧ Let's say it's September. When you look at your patient records, you'll be able to see quickly that anyone who doesn't have a current year sticker must be past due since it's already the ninth month of the year.
- ✧ Pull all those records and place them in a separate file alphabetically.
- ✧ Determine the number of staff members who can help make these calls and the amount of time they can dedicate each day. This works well when the staff has organizational time (see pages 5-14) or when the dentist is on vacation or attending continuing education.
- ✧ Document the results of the phone conversations you have with each patient. After a reactivation call is completed, record the name of the patient, whether appointed or not, and, if inactivated, the reasons for the patient leaving the practice.
- ✧ Report the results of these calls in the aggregate at your next regular staff meeting. An example, "Last month, I called sixty-seven inactive patients. Of these, twenty-eight made appointments, three left for [this reason], two left for [that reason]," and so on. The charts are either re-filed to the active or inactive filing areas determined by the results of the call. If a patient wishes to be placed in an inactive file, the dentist should review his or her chart before it is filed.

Recare Appointments and Staff Incentives
Some doctors find it beneficial to offer an incentive for staff who successfully schedule these patients, perhaps something like $5 for each reactivated patient and $10 for any new patients (family members). Incentives make the job of telemarketing inactive patients more fun. By introducing a little friendly competition, incentives also build a sense of teamwork. In addition, it simply makes good business sense to pay your staff to help you build your practice. Finally, the cost of these incentives is very low compared to what a new or reactivated patient will be worth to the practice over time.

CHAPTER 9

Dynamic Practice Guidelines

THERE ARE ESSENTIALLY TWO WAYS TO MANAGE A DENTAL OFFICE: with policies—what I call practice guidelines—and without them. Without practice guidelines, patients decide when and if they are coming and when and if they will pay. They are quite literally running the practice. The staff is in chaos, without boundaries and uncertain of their roles and responsibilities or the appropriate ways to respond to the many situations that arise in the normal press of business. The staff members also feel unimportant and unappreciated. Stress levels are high. Production is low.

I've personally seen some pretty burnt out dental practices in which the doctor at age forty is ready to find another profession, and very often one of the primary reasons is the fact that the doctor's working fifty to sixty hours a week in a chaotic environment where the patients determine when the doctor will see them and employees create their own job descriptions and policies.

With practice guidelines that are enforced with fairness and consistency, an office runs full tilt on all eight cylinders. Staff members are happy and motivated. Each person has what I call "role clarity"—a clear sense of their responsibilities, importance, and accountabilities within the practice.

Patients' high expectations are met, they are satisfied with the treatment they receive in the office—both in and out of the chair—and they respect and abide by the office policies and procedures. Payments are made on time and patients are satisfied, the environment is happy, order prevails. Stress is low and production is high. Policies provide structure and predictability, two qualities essential to a healthy, positive work environment in which everyone knows what's expected of them and success is a set of clear targets for the practice and each individual in it.

Practice guidelines make success seamless and effortless. A lack of guidelines ensures that success will elude the practice year after year and make daily operations a struggle.

Practice guidelines are needed in an office for everything from the office dress code to collections policies to personal days.

To make practice guidelines worthwhile, that is, enforceable and valuable, two rules apply: 1) they must be in writing, and 2) everyone—including and sometimes especially the dentist—must adhere to them. As the leader of the practice, the dentist must "walk the talk" of the practice guidelines manual by setting an impeccable example in his choices and actions every day. If he doesn't, he can rest assured the staff will follow his poor example. Every organization reflects the personality and work ethic of its leader—for better or worse—and a dental practice is no exception.

By the way, I refer to practice guidelines instead of policies because I believe the word "guideline" conveys a small measure of flexibility: a guideline can be bent but never broken.

To make it easy to use, I've organized this chapter into a round-up of short passages that describe policies I believe are most essential to the success of every dental practice...dynamic dentistry in action!

Discuss these policies as a team...add, delete, and otherwise edit as needed to make them reflect the needs of your unique practice and its patients.

There are two broad categories: guidelines that influence how patients must be handled and guidelines that manage employees.

Remember...

Practice guidelines are not set in stone. Every practice has the right to change these guidelines from time to time, based on business needs or changes in competitive practices.

The keys to an easy and seamless transition to a new guideline are:

1. Analyzing the need for the change.
2. Developing the new guideline and adjusting any corresponding policies as needed.
3. Putting the new guideline in writing.
4. Communicating the change to the people inside and outside the practice that will be affected by it.
5. Providing those affected by the change with sufficient lead time before the change is effective.

Operations and Patient Relations

Collections

Firm office policies mean low accounts receivable. Create policies for handling:

1. New patients and emergencies
2. Criteria for granting financial options
3. Cases involving lab work
4. Insurance co-payments
5. Insurance deductibles
6. Fee presentation
7. Interest charges
8. Statement dates
9. Credit card policies
10. Courtesies
11. Senior citizen courtesies

Emergencies

Far too often emergency patients are turned away from dental practices at the front desk because the doctor and team have never established firm guidelines for how the practice will handle emergencies. Emergency patients are essential to the growth of your practice.

See Chapter 6 for detailed guidance on handling emergencies effectively and efficiently in your practice.

Interrupting the Dentist

✧ In a well organized practice, the front desk person or schedul ing coordinator has been given a short list of the people and situations for which the doctor will take chairside interruptions. These may include family emergencies, other doctors, and long-distance calls.

✧ The staff should never announce the calls chairside. Patients will feel they are less than top priority. Instead, the person taking the call should write notes, use a light signaling system, or computer messaging for those few interruptions that require the doctor to leave the patient.

✧ For those calls that can be handled, the scheduling coordinator should say, "The doctor is in with a patient. How may I help you?" or "May I take a number? How long will you be at this number?"

Handling Patients

✧ Keeping patients waiting for more than ten minutes, no matter what the reason, is detrimental to practice success and growth. Strive to keep patient wait time at ten minutes or less.

✧ Be certain employees are prepared to handle a wide variety of patient situations such as the following:

Situation: A patient doesn't want to pay the co-pay.

What to do: Mr. Brown, I know we've billed you in the past, but effective three months ago, we are accepting co-payments at the time of treatment to avoid the need to hire another full-time employee. This would have meant increasing our fees twenty percent, which we preferred not to do.

Situation: A patient is rude.
What to do: Kill them with kindness! Some people are not happy and their goal in life is to be a joy robber of others. Stay calm when dealing with rude patients. Be firm yet friendly in your approach and realize that two percent of your patients will simply never be pleased…and you must stop trying to please them.

Situation: A patient had no intention of paying today at time of service.
What to do: Reinforce the office guidelines that payments are due at the time of service. Let them know that you also accept credit cards. Then give them a walkout statement with a stamped envelope and tell them to please put the check in the mail tomorrow.

Situation: A hygiene patient doesn't want to accept treatment unless it's covered by insurance.
What to do: Remind the patient that insurance covers basic preventive and basic restorative care and ninety-five percent of all adults need more than basic dentistry.

Situation: A patient is habitually more than fifteen minutes late.
What to do: Schedule the patient at one time and write the time on their appointment card for twenty minutes earlier. They will arrive on time every appointment.

Situation: A patient refuses to floss or even brush their teeth on a regular basis.
What to do: Remind the patient that they must be accountable to having a clean and healthy mouth. We as dental professionals can help them with their mission, but is totally up to them whether they wish to retain their teeth through adulthood.

Employee Relations

Guidelines give employees a sense of structure and security. Specific guidelines need to be established and communicated to employees for:

- commitment to patients
- financial success targets
- standards and expectations
- emphasis on teamwork

They should also understand the office's practice guidelines regarding:

- smoking
- personal phone calls
- dress code
- sick/vacation/personal time (amount of paid time off for which each employee is eligible, as well as the process for requesting vacation and personal days)
- lunch breaks
- staff education and training seminars
- performance reviews
- salary increases

You might also consider creating guidelines for bereavement leave for the death of an immediate family member, as well as for jury duty.

Dynamic practice guidelines support the success and growth of a dental practice because they are crystal clear, written, given to every employee on the very first day of their employment, and followed equally by everyone in the practice. This is how a business—any business—avoids burnout and reaches breakthrough levels of success.

CHAPTER 10

Marketing Suggestions

THE WORD MARKETING OFTEN CONFUSES PEOPLE. SOME USE IT synonymously with sales, but marketing is much more than that, although sales promotion is part of marketing. Some think of marketing as public relations. Again, public relations is essential, but only a part of marketing. Creating an identity for your dental practice is another essential component of your marketing activities as is engaging the enthusiastic support of your employees to serve as goodwill ambassadors within your community.

Here's a useful definition from *The Marketing Glossary* by Mark Clemente: marketing is "the complex, interrelated series of activities involved in creating products and services, promoting their existence and attributes, and making them physically available to identified target buyers. Marketing is comprised of four distinct processes:

1. developing the product or service
2. establishing a price for it
3. communicating information about it through various...channels,
4. coordinating its distribution..."

This may sound complex, but marketing for a dental practice is primarily a combination of one or more of the following:

- ✧ print and sometimes radio or even cable TV advertising (Note that the State Board of Dentistry must critique ads and brochures for dental practices before they're published. Mailing lists must also be approved.)
- ✧ direct mail solicitations
- ✧ various activities that ensure the dentist's and the practice's image within the community, including the business community

To truly complete this list, I must add a few things we don't ordinarily think of as part of marketing, but which are actually essential to it:

- ✧ staff and doctor's attitudes
- ✧ the quality of the recare system
- ✧ the overall appearance of the office
- ✧ the practice's logo and its use on business cards, appointment cards, letterhead, etc.

I've discussed the essential importance of staff attitude in a number of places in previous chapters. When it comes to marketing, engaged, motivated employees who enjoy being in a caring profession and believe in the expertise of the dentist and hygienist are irreplaceable. They become goodwill ambassadors within your patient base and the community at large.

As I discussed in detail in Chapter 8, your recare system is the heart of ongoing patient flow to the practice.

Remember that patients judge the unknown (dentistry) by the known (the appearance of the office and its surroundings). The modern dental office should not reflect the starched professionalism of the past. Today's practices need to be warm, friendly, yet professional places that patients enjoy visiting. Adults as well as children need to feel welcome the minute they walk through the door.

I truly believe in the "open concept" for the business arena. The greeter needs to be able to see the entire reception area so she can see patients arriving. If she is on the phone when a patient arrives, she can always smile and nod to acknowledge the person's presence and indicate she'll only be a moment. It's best to have the front desk in an open setting, with no barriers between the staff and patients.

The patients' restroom should be the most beautifully decorated room in the office—at least as nice as the guest bathroom of a home. Think about how much money is spent to make the guest bath at home perfect yet so few guests ever use it. On the other hand, approximately twenty patients per day visit your office restroom, yet many times corners are cut on this small but significant item. It amazes me how many practices still have the institutional towel box with white or brown scratchy paper towels for the patients' use. Would you have these in a guest bath at home? A "community terrycloth towel" is not the answer, but how about soft, colorful disposable towels in a nice tray. It's the same difference as having lunch at a family steakhouse with plastic trays and bare tables versus the country club with nice linens! Your patients are like guests in your home. Treat them that way and watch your practice flourish.

I also recommend nice plumbing fixtures, paint or nice wallpaper, marble or nice tile on the floor, paintings or pictures, silk flowers, or other decorative items. For the patients' comfort, there should be mouthwash samples, disposable toothbrushes, and floss. A tray of hand lotion, hairspray, and colognes add a welcome touch. Many cosmetic companies will furnish businesses with samples of their products for commercial use as a form of advertising. Your local Mary Kay distributor will be glad to give samples of lipstick, etc.

In your reception area, improve the quality of reading material. (As we know, the caliber of reading materials suggests the educational level you feel your patients have.) Place nice bound cookbooks in the room along with recipe cards imprinted with the doctor's name, address, and telephone number at the top. Patients who wait can copy the recipes they like. Add plants and small containers of potpourri to the reception room to give it life and a pleasant fragrance.

The office must be spotlessly clean. The pride we have in our personal surroundings reflects the pride we have in the work we do. Everyone can and should share in an effort to have a shining, clean office. The office should be dusted and vacuumed daily, sinks should be polished at all times, and trash receptacles should never be within view of the patient. I have heard patients say, "I judge the sterility of the instruments by how clean and tidy the entire office is." Would your office pass this patient test?

A patient once left a practice because the same dirty cotton roll was on the floor in front of the sink two weeks in a row. She decided, appropriately, that they did not clean very thoroughly.

Take a look at the office from the patient's vantage point. Sit in the dental chairs and in the reception room at least once a week and look around. In a reclined position in the dental chair, do you see dead bugs in the light or ceiling tiles that need to be replaced? In the reception room, do you see dust on picture frames, chipped paint on woodwork, and outdated, torn magazines? Patients may not know for years how great your dentistry is, but they immediately know how they feel in your office.

The outer appearance of the office, the street location, the sign on the street or building, and the facility itself form the patient's very first impressions of the practice. If the building is attractive and the location is good, potential patients will note this. When they need a dentist, they'll remember, "I liked the looks of that dental office on Maple Street, and it is close to work."

With respect to office locations, bear in mind that a dental office is much like a restaurant. Three things are important to success: location, exposure, and area. Location is a very good predictor of the type of clientele that will come to the office. It's important for dentists to know which types of patients they want to attract when selecting the office location. Exposure is essential to practice success. Highly traveled areas with good street exposure bring the best new-patient results.

The exterior sign on the building should reflect the quality of dentistry being offered. It is the office's calling card on the street. The sign should display the practice logo and match the building in design. For instance, contemporary offices should have a contemporary sign, traditional offices should have a traditional sign, and colonial offices should have a colonial sign. (Some municipalities have codes regarding signs and their designs. Building owners also want some say in the appearance of outside areas. Check with each of these before investing in signage for the practice.)

Taken together, all these factors send messages—visually and/or verbally—that make an impression and strengthen the practice's identity in the eyes of the patient.

By the Numbers

Naturally, the point of marketing is to help the practice grow by attracting a steady flow of new patients while continuing to provide existing patients with superior care. How does a practice set targets for an influx of new patients?

Some offices feel they have a healthy number of new patients at twelve per month. Other offices have no idea how many new patients they have monthly because they don't keep score. The ideal number of new patients is difficult to determine because it depends on the type of services provided and the existing patient base. If a dentist is losing more than 200 hygiene visits per month because there is no room in the hygiene schedule to get them in, why would they continuously take forty to sixty new patients per month? If a practice does complete mouth rehab dentistry at $20,000 to $40,000 per case, they can get by on very few new patients (fewer than ten per month).

In a highly transient area of the country such as a military setting, the new patient number may be thirty to forty per month while in a more stable area, twenty new patients are plenty. A new dentist with a nonexistent patient base may in fact welcome forty to fifty new patients per month as every patient is new.

There are many variables involved. It is truly sad to watch an existing practice decline. New patient numbers are below ten, patients in the telemarketing calls inform the staff member they will not be back, and the dentist reduces the number of hygiene days because the hygiene schedule is not full. These "free fall" practices are normally close to rock bottom by the time they realize they are losing more patients than they are retaining. It is often impossible to get the numbers up and the practice back on track before the cry for help goes out.

What causes these types of dramatic practice changes:

1. Abrupt changes in policies without the staff being properly trained to present the changes in a positive manner.
2. Lack of focus by the leader. I.e., Being distracted to build a home or office, outside businesses, getting married/divorced, a personal tragedy, being in debt with no end in sight, or total burnout.
3. Rumors in the community of health problems or other damaging personal issues.
4. Not "minding the store" monthly by asking for monitors and not knowing how to be a consultant to one's own practice by interpreting the numbers to identify hidden management problems before they become destructive.
5. Not staying current with techniques, technology, materials, which "ages" your practice.

Create a Set of Marketing Messages

Develop a set of marketing messages to use in all your promotional materials. Some examples:

- ✧ "community-oriented"
- ✧ "preventive dentistry with a cosmetic flair"
- ✧ "patient-centered"
- ✧ "promptness is our goal"
- ✧ "state-of-the-art technology"
- ✧ "conscientious, well-trained staff"
- ✧ "preventive, restorative, cosmetic"

Your goal is to use these messages to develop an identity in the community and among current and future patients. What do you stand for? What sets your practice apart?

These messages comprise a complete and distinct identity for your practice. For example, Linda Miles Associates' identity is "Dentistry's Leading Practice and Staff Development Company" through which I strive to communicate high quality, responsiveness, and many years of expertise in the dental field. Also, I always include my photograph, through which I want to communicate my high level of involvement and personal service. Every promotion I create reinforces this identity, and I do not waver from it. Our website is www.dentalmanagementu.com. Our other domain sites include DMU Seminars, DMU Conferences, DMU Products, etc. Anyone looking up the words "dental management" will find us.

In creating these messages, determine the target group(s) to which you want to appeal (children, young parents, middle-aged business people, workers, and/or senior citizens), since your messages will need to appeal to the groups you're trying to attract to the practice. This is called the "rifle" approach versus the "shotgun" approach to marketing.

Three Essential Factors

Two factors are at the heart of all successful marketing activities: repetition and consistency. People must see the same sales promotion messages consistently over a period of time in order to know that your dental practice provides state-of-the-art, high quality dentistry and is dedicated to patients and to the community. Your practice brochure must include the same messages you might use in a print advertisement, the dentist must use these messages in a talk at a community gathering, and you should include them in a "Welcome to Our Practice" letter to new patients.

Clearly, the same messages repeated with consistency will help you build a base of recognition within the community needed to help your practice succeed and grow. Each time someone sees your practice name and logo, it registers and eventually becomes a conscious desire to try out the practice. Thus, your ads, brochures, newsletters, etc. should look and sound similar, reinforcing the same image and message over and over.

A third essential factor applies most especially to the marketing efforts of dental practices: class and professionalism. Don't be too casual or familiar in your sales promotion messages and approach. I often advise clients to stay away from techniques like coupons or excessively cute advertising since these do not convey class and professionalism. Remember, everything that leaves the office is a reflection of what goes on inside it.

Two-Thirds Internal; One-Third External

The formula for successful marketing of a dental practice is sixty-five percent internal and thirty-five percent external. Internal marketing refers to promoting the practice by the employees who work in it. It also refers to efforts aimed at encouraging referrals from the practice's existing patient base—make each visit an experience your patients will talk happily about—and need I mention, consistent preventive care of those patients as needed (see Chapter 8 for more). External marketing refers of course to reaching out to the community, potential patients, and even specialists with whom your practice works.

Why this balance? Two key reasons: first, your staff is your sales force. Much of your marketing energy should be focused on them because when they are helped to feel positive about the practice and its ability to help patients, they radiate this confidence and patients sense it and want to come back for more. It's a self-perpetuating cycle of positive energy and practice growth. Second, it's less expensive to keep an existing patient than to get a new one. So doing all you can to keep patients happy and well cared for is a must.

First Things

Develop a Logo

I strongly recommend that you invest in a professionally designed and produced logo for your practice. Hire a graphic artist to draw a logo or give the assignment to an advertising agency.

The logo should be on everything that leaves your office and represents the practice, including your listing in the Yellow Pages, your business cards, appointment cards, correspondence, and the sign outside your office. Bear in mind as you're developing this logo that your practice should be associated with a graphic image that is sophisticated, tasteful, and distinctive (not a dancing tooth!) and you're in the business of saving and enhancing teeth, not extracting them!

A logo identifies the practice and provides important visibility when used correctly on everything that represents your office. It serves to reinforce the practice's image and ensure its visibility within the community and the dental profession. It also suggests a high level of professionalism and business savvy. Taken together, all these messages convey that your practice offers serious, state-of-the-art dentistry and that your office provides the highest levels of patient service.

Remember that consistency counts. The logo must be used in the same way across all communication channels. For instance, if the image is blue and green, it should always be shown in blue and green, not brown and orange on some pieces and blue and green on others. If it includes a graphic image such as a sphere, it should always include that image as a three-dimensional sphere, not a circle. This may seem minor, but it is absolutely not. To get the real repetition value out of having a logo, it must be used with the utmost consistency. It must always have a uniform look and feel.

The "Gentle Dental" and the "We Cater to Cowards" messages that have been around for thirty years are dated and have a seventies feel, not a new millennium look. Then again, some practitioners give those two slogans credit for making their practices successful and would not think of changing them. As I've said before, one size does not fit all practices in marketing or anything else. Decide what type of patients and practice you want in three years and build your marketing plan around it.

Focus on Patient Education

One of the greatest marketing tools at your disposal is patient education. I personally don't believe that through TV and radio media the public should know more about personal hygiene products and laxatives than they do about dental care, but this is generally the case. The good news is that you can use this fact as a marketing opportunity by including patient education in your sales promotion efforts.

This may include community talks given by the dentist at community gatherings from Rotary and Chamber of Commerce meetings to garden clubs and business group meetings, where lawyers, bankers, realtors, and insurance agents convene. Create a talk for bankers and investment planners about how your smile improves your face value. Develop a half-hour talk on cosmetic dentistry to deliver to the community. Show before and after slides. Women's groups are particularly fertile ground for community talks as seventy-five percent of dental care is influenced by the female consumer.

Talk Up Dentistry

Emphasize the wonderful decision the patient's made to have whatever procedure they are sitting in the chair for. Talk up dentistry. Talk up the dentist and the hygienist. One of the greatest marketing tools that you could have is a staff that continually says things like, "I work for the greatest dentist in the whole world," "I probably have the best job in this town," and "I love what I do."

Handle Patient Referrals Like Rare Jewels

Patient referrals are the lifeblood of your practice growth, and each one is a vote of confidence from a patient sending his or her friends and family to you. It's good form and smart business to make the effort to thank patients for their trust and belief in the practice's ability to take good care of the people they send to the practice.

Here's how to thank someone and make your office "referral-friendly":

1. Include a question about who referred the patient on the initial patient information form.

2. When the referred patient gives you the name of a referring patient, always say something nice about the referring party. For example, "Joan Black is one of my favorite patients. I always look forward to her visits" or "Joan Black refers such nice people to us." These compliments always go back to the referral source.

3. Ask for referrals on a regular basis and develop a "we care" referral card that is kept in the treatment rooms as well as at the desk. Have it say something like, "If you have friends, relatives, or co-

workers who do not have a personal dentist, please let them know we would love to see them."

4. Send a thank-you to each referring patient: a handwritten, informal note, for instance. If a patient is especially loyal and refers several new patients, the office may want to do something special. Flowers are nice for women, fruit baskets are appreciated by both sexes. For either men or women, lunch for two or theatre tickets are nice ways to say thank you. Consider gift certificates for movies, lunch, ice cream, car washes, etc. Local businesses enjoy being part of your appreciation scheme. They and their employees also become potential patients as the word spreads.

> Patients like to feel special. When new dentists open practices, they have time to make their patients feel this way. But after a while, dentists and staff often commit the mistake of spending extra time and effort making new patients welcome while treating their returning patients as just so many warm bodies in the chairs. The entire dental team should always strive to make all patients feel "new-patient special."

Create a marketing plan for the year by following these steps:

1. Develop a budget for the year.
2. Determine the target group(s) to which you want to appeal, one group per month or quarter.
3. Select one marketing strategy at a time to try to attract each target group, factoring in each month's marketing budget.
4. Monitor the effectiveness of each marketing strategy by asking every new patient how they heard about the practice and enter their response into the computer. Discuss these results at your regular staff meetings, and make adjustments in your marketing program accordingly. Most software packages include this tracking system and if yours doesn't, it could soon become an update at your request.

One note: No matter what internal or external marketing the office chooses to implement, be sure to ask for the staff's input on marketing ideas. When everyone's involved, marketing always has more momentum and energy, which makes it more effective.

Marketing Strategies

What follows are a number of marketing ideas. Select a few or more that match the personality and marketing goals of your practice, and give them a try.

General Dentistry

For All Patients...

- ✧ Send a "Welcome to Our Practice" letter or brochure introducing the doctor, practice philosophy, and staff prior to the patient's first visit. It also is nice to include an appointment card, a map of the office location, and the patient registration form that will need to be completed at the first appointment.
- ✧ Send a card or letter stating, "Thank you for selecting our office... We enjoyed getting to know you and look forward to seeing you in the future..." after the patient's first visit.
- ✧ Offer twenty-four hour availability. An answering service or a call forwarding or answering device with remote control enables the dentist to be available twenty-four hours a day. In building a new practice, this availability is essential. In an established practice, it is good public relations.
- ✧ Send an e-newsletter. A newsletter should be a team effort with each member of the team contributing a short capsule on their part of the practice. The hygienist may write something about "Hygiene Tips," "Sugar-Free Recipes," etc. The financial coordinator may write an"Insurance Update" or about the exciting financial options the practice now offers. Someone else may do the "Children's Corner" or "On the Road Again" (a list of the

continuing education courses the staff and doctor have attended), or "Patient Awareness Tips." If you have a specialty practice, e-mail the newsletter to general dentists in the area. At dental meetings, ask other practice personnel who create e-newsletters to add your office to their mailing list.

✧ Call injected patients in the evening to see how well they are doing after their visit that day. Never say, "I'm calling to see if you're having problems" or you'll be on the phone all night! Simply say that you want to be certain they're doing all right, or you're calling to see how well they're doing.

✧ Provide business cards for the staff. Team members cannot be enthused about "their" office if they do not feel important. Staff business cards can be a great marketing tool if used as intended. If each staff member has a personal business card, giving them away becomes a matter of habit. The staff should take them everywhere they go. For example, when staff go to the dry cleaners or on any other personal errand and the service person asks "May I have your name and telephone number?", the staff member can pull out a card and leave it. At banks and grocery stores, when the clerks ask for identification, the staff member can give the necessary identification and leave a card as well. Their name and title are in the middle with: "Office of: Dr.____________" at the bottom. Using cards effectively is a habit everyone can develop.

✧ Send baby gifts to new mothers. Anytime there is a new baby in a family, a prospective new patient has been born. Giving a baby toothbrush, a teething ring, or some other type of baby item is another way of saying "We care."

✧ Give certificates for new parents. Send certificates to new parents saying, "Congratulations on your new arrival. This entitles you to your child's first dental exam when he or she is two years old. Compliments of Dr.______ & Staff."

✧ Place pamphlets on baby bottle syndrome and pregnancy

gingivitis in the reception area of OB/GYN practices.

✧ Offer to serve as the dentist for retirement and nursing homes.

✧ If you have hours before 8:00 a.m. or after 5:00 p.m., publicize them as "executive" and "convenient hours."

✧ Offer a complimentary prophylaxis and exam to couples who are recently engaged (a pre-nuptial prophy).

✧ Offer a ten percent courtesy if patients agree to be on your Special Call List for short notice appointments.

✧ Be respectful of your patient's time. If they are kept waiting, apologize and offer movie, car wash, or ice cream certificates.

✧ Give portrait studio certificates to patients who have received extensive cosmetic treatment.

✧ Take before and after photos of extensive treatments.

✧ Place an atlas of modern cosmetic and restorative dentistry in the reception area and in each treatment room. If the clinical staff must leave the treatment room they can say, "Mrs. Phillips, while I check on your x-rays/get the doctor, let me show you these before and after cosmetic cases we are so proud of!" A before and after photo is an incredible teaching aid.

✧ When dismissing the patient, remember to invite their family, friends, and coworkers.

✧ Offer complimentary prophylaxis to new or current patients who have successfully quit smoking...New patients should be referred by a quit smoking organization such as the American Cancer Society or a hospital in your area.

✧ Provide washable blankets to cover patients who may get cool during treatment.

✧ Offer tea, coffee, and juice to patients when they arrive early. A refreshment center in one part of the reception area gives your office a first-class, "red carpet" feeling.

✧ Present imprinted golf tees to patients who enjoy golf.

✧ Present cosmetic makeover certificates to patients who have completed cosmetic treatment. (Your local department stores' cosmetic departments can help you arrange this.)

✧ Have toothbrushes and floss imprinted with your name and telephone number for recare patients.

✧ Sponsor dental poster contests at schools.

✧ Obtain new homeowners' names from real estate listings and send a letter or brochure introducing your practice.

✧ Send a card or gift to ill or hospitalized patients.

✧ Provide pre-stamped stationery in your reception area so patients can write personal notes while they wait.

✧ Create a "Patient Happenings" or VIP (Very Important Patient) wall with framed news or photographs of patients.

✧ Place an album in your reception area that contains thank you notes from patients.

✧ Rent a booth at a bridal show with before and after cosmetic whitening cases. A sign should read, "On your wedding day we want your smile to be whiter and brighter."

✧ Place an ad in a specialty publication such as a newspaper that goes out to military households declaring a coming Military Appreciation Month to invite military families to the practice. Place a similar ad in a school publication regarding how much the practice appreciates educational personnel: "You build the future of our world." Make the next month Medical Staff Appreciation, and so on.

For Children…

- ✧ Have a children's corner or kiddy theatre in your reception area with favorite CDs and videos to keep small children entertained while they wait.
- ✧ Give away a Tooth Fairy Membership Kit. Included is a tooth brush, a tooth chest for lost primary teeth, a tooth fairy bravery badge, and other assorted prizes.
- ✧ Give a prescription for a free milkshake. Every time a child patient leaves the office, write a special prescription on a preprinted child-like prescription pad. Arrange ahead of time with your local ice cream store to do this. "Rx: Dispense one free milkshake (any flavor) to _____for being a great patient today. Signed: Dr.________________________."
- ✧ Give out balloons, stickers, rings, and other prizes. Children love prizes and look forward to their visit to the dentist if they get to dig through the toy chest or put a nickel (provided by the office) into the prize machine.
- ✧ Offer a $1,000 scholarship to a student patient who goes into dental hygiene, dental assisting, or pre-dental. The doctor should present the scholarship and have photos taken for the paper.

Specialists

Encourage referrals from other practitioners with these marketing techniques:

- ✧ Communicate with referring doctors through e-mail for patients' clinical updates. Ask them to enter notes into patient records electronically or print a hard copy for patient records.
- ✧ Treat the referring doctor and staff for reduced fees. "I want you to feel so good about us that you will recommend us to your patients, friends, and family without hesitation."
- ✧ If the patient does not want to go back to the referring doctor, communicate your concern. "Can I come by and see you at the

end of the day? I have a problem I need to discuss with you. I need your help." Or, "Your patient does not want to come back to you. I need your help." This lets the referring doctor know it is not your choice, but the patient's.

- ✧ Pediatric and orthodontic practices can have an open house and invite patients and their friends. Have music and provide healthy snacks. Select a theme, i.e., Halloween Party, Fourth of July, Back-to-School, etc.
- ✧ Compliment the skills of the referring doctor to the patient. Inform the referring doctor of positive remarks his/her patient communicated to you regarding his/her clinical skills or his or her practice in general.
- ✧ Offer complimentary consultations and evaluations to new patients referred by a current patient.
- ✧ When the patient is checking out, have your appointment coordinator call the referring doctor's appointment coordinator to schedule the patient's alternating recare visits and restorative/operative care. Your appointment coordinator is actually making the appointments for the patients while they are still in the office. This keeps alternating preventive care appointments on par as an added service benefit to the patients.
- ✧ Send a questionnaire to referring doctors asking:
  a. How can we work better with your office?
  b. Concerns or comments?
- ✧ Have an open house buffet lunch for referring doctors and their staffs at your office or a local restaurant.
- ✧ Host a practice management or clinical seminar by providing a speaker and inviting all your referring practices to attend as your guests. (See our website Speakers Bureau under Speaking Consultant Network (www.dentalmanagementU.com) for a list of recommended speakers.)
- ✧ Invite referring doctors to attend continuing education seminars as your guests.

- ✧ Support the treatment plan of the referring doctor and the objectives of the case ahead of time. "Send me your intentions before I see your patient so I can support your treatment plan."
- ✧ Help new general practitioners get started.
- ✧ Give referring doctors a subscription to your specialty journal.
- ✧ Hold a monthly two-hour luncheon for your "Top Twelve" referring practices. During lunch, have the clinical staff sit with the clinical staff from the referring practices, the business staff sit with the business staff of the referring practices, and the specialist sit with the dentist. Conduct a twenty-minute informal mini-seminar on your specialty topics.
- ✧ Send unique thank-you gifts that can be enjoyed by the entire office.
- ✧ Send special cards to your referring doctors and staff at Thanksgiving time. Enclose a photograph of you and your staff.
- ✧ Distribute your patient information brochures to your referring practices. Attach your business card and directions to your practice.
- ✧ Offer to pay the dues for your staff members to join the ADAA and ADHA. Networking with staff from other offices can increase referrals.
- ✧ Send patients back to referring doctor, stressing the importance of completing treatment.
- ✧ Offer to be a guest speaker at the referring doctor's next staff meeting. During your lecture, compliment the referring doctor's dentistry.
- ✧ Take the referring dentist and his/her spouse to dinner or send a gift certificate to a nice restaurant.
- ✧ Create and send a monthly e-newsletter to patients and referring practices.

CHAPTER 11

This Could Be the Start of Something Big!

WELL, HERE WE ARE, TEN CHAPTERS LATER, READY TO WRAP UP. We've covered a lot of ground on our journey together. I hope you've gained a great deal from this book, and that you feel prepared to create your own dynamic dental practice. I hope too that your vision of what's possible for your practice is clear: excellence, achievement, increased production, a growing patient base, a joyful, healthy workplace, a thriving business.

This truly can be the start of something big. Just how big?

To give you a hint of where I think the best dental practices are headed, let me leave you with my vision of the future of dentistry, a future filled with dynamic dental practices...

> Sally Rogers—dental patient from the not-too-distant future—walks into a foyer, illuminated with soft lights, an elegant Oriental rug on the floor.
>
> As she approaches the front desk, she is greeted warmly by a staff member who says, "Good morning, Ms. Rogers, and welcome to Dr. Williams' office. Please relax for a few minutes in the reception area. We're just about ready for you."

She finds a comfortable armchair, listens to the classical music, enjoys the beautiful artwork—perhaps an original watercolor or tapestry—and reads the latest issue of Architectural Digest.

Within five minutes, a bright, smiling, very professional dental assistant named Joann calls her name and escorts her to a treatment room where Joann explains the day's procedure and answers a few of Sally's questions. Dr. Williams is in momentarily to begin the procedure. Dr. Williams and Joann work efficiently, but without rushing, and they chat lightly during the procedure. It's clear they respect one another and enjoy working together.

After the procedure, Dr. Williams says, "Sally, I'm going to leave you in Joann's very capable hands. She'll take care of you from here." He continues his day with the next patient.

Joann conducts some post-treatment education, then tells Sally to relax for a few moments while she enters Sally's treatment information, schedules her next appointment chairside, and then escorts her to Gina, the practice's financial coordinator. Joann greets Gina with a friendly tone that demonstrates these coworkers genuinely like one another, introduces Sally, and hands Sally's record over to Gina with the following statement, "Sally, it was great seeing you today. I look forward to your next visit. Gina will process your insurance now, and she'll give you your receipt for today's visit."

"How are you feeling, Sally?" Gina asks, genuinely interested.

"Oh, okay. A little numb," says Sally.

Gina smiles, understanding. "Well, I won't make you talk too much, then," she says. "Sally, the fee for today is two seventy-five. Will that be cash, check, or bank card?"

"Check," says Sally, whereupon she writes the check for payment in full, thanks Gina, and leaves, feeling well cared for and fully satisfied.

Dr. Williams' practice functions on all eight cylinders. Accounts receivable are low; production is increasing steadily. The schedule has very few gaps. Cancellations are uncommon and quickly filled by the scheduling coordinator, whose creative strategies for filling the sched-

> ule include using her short notice call list and pending lists consistently rather than moving already scheduled patients. The hygienist practices assisted hygiene to treat up to fifteen patients each day with her own full-time, designated assistant.

Why has everything gone so well, so smoothly? By now of course you know there are many reasons, specifically guidelines and strategies in place, that make this practice run efficiently with an air of calm professionalism. You also know that what underlies each and every one of these guidelines and strategies are two words: attitude and communication.

The dentist sets the tone for the office with the practice and the staff. It is an attitude of inclusion. Everyone is part of the team; team members know their roles and have the independence to fulfill them and the accountability that accompanies it. That attitude permeates the entire office and every aspect of patient interaction.

As part of that inclusion, a spirit of open and positive communication exists among all staff members. Regular staff meetings enable the team to discuss what's working and what needs fixing and provide a forum for everyone to listen and be heard. The conversation among staff members is always positive, affirming what's working well and dealing with criticisms behind closed doors.

Perhaps most important, everyone, whether a staff member or a patient, knows they're being treated equally and fairly.

Depending on the state of your practice today, this may be a short or a long journey, but one, I promise, worth embarking upon. I wish you the very best in building the dynamic dental practice of your dreams. Please do let this be the start of something big—very big—for you.

I'd enjoy hearing about your experiences along the way. Feel free to contact me at www.dentalmanagementu.com. For a complete list of seminars, products, and services, you may reach me at 800-922-0866.

Appendix A

At several points in this book, I have identified words and phrases that should and should not be used in a dynamic dental practice. The underlying concepts behind these words and phrases are positive, easy-to-understand speech.

You may want to photocopy and post the following lists so staff members can refer to them often.

Dynamic Patient Communications

Instead of...	**Use...**
Waiting room	Reception room
Operatory	Treatment room
Private office	Consultation area
Full mouth series	Necessary x-rays
Study models	Diagnostic models
Rehabilitation	Complete dentistry
Work	Treatment or dentistry
Cavities	Decay
Fillings	Restoration
Temporary filling	Sedative restoration
Remove/Pull	Extraction
Simple	Uncomplicated
Recall	Recare
Grind the tooth	Prepare the tooth
Partials	Partial denture
Baby teeth	Primary or deciduous teeth
My girl	My assistant
Price or charge	Fee

Instead of...	**Use...**
Bill	Statement
Would you like/ How do you plan to pay?	Your fee is _____. Will that be cash, check, or bank card?
Payment arrangements	Financial options
Pay for	Take care of
Contract or note	Agreement
Cost	Investment
Your fee is $165 dollars.	Your fee is one-sixty-five.
Three hundred twenty-seven dollars	Three twenty-seven
I suggest	I recommend
The doctor would like	The doctor recommends
Discount	Courtesy
Professional discount	Professional courtesy
Old patient	Patient of record; former patient
Check-up	Thorough examination
Syringe/Needle	Call by color
Pain/hurt	Discomfort
When would you like to come in?	Do you prefer morning or afternoons?
Cancellation	Change in schedule
Old filling	Restoration that has outlived it's usefulness
I'm calling to remind you about your appointment.	We look forward to seeing you tomorrow at noon.
May I ask who's calling?	May I tell the doctor who is calling?

Instead of…	Use…
Cleaning the room	Preparing the treatment area
Would you like to come in?	Ms. Jones, the doctor is ready to see you.
Who's calling please?	Dr. Smith is with a patient; how may I help you?
Do you want to leave a message?	How may I help you?
He's booked. He can't see you until____.	The doctor's schedule is filled today, but he can see you at _____.
Thank you for calling.	Thank you for calling, (and their name).
I'm sorry, I can't fit you in today.	How soon can you be here?
The doctor is running late.	The doctor has had an interruption in his schedule.
Remind	Looking forward to seeing you at___.
Denture adjustment	Observation appointment
Do you understand…?	How do you feel about…?
Drill	High speed or low speed
Chisel, forceps	By number
Grind	Reshape
Open wide	Open big (to a child)
Business office	Administrative office
Call the doctor by first name in front of patient	Dr. Smith
Spit	Rinse
Old patient	Patient of record
Receptionist	Scheduling or business coordinator
Office manager	Practice administrator

Dynamic Communication Strategies	
On the Phone	
Instead of:	"Good morning, I mean afternoon. Dr. Smith's office."
Use:	"Thank you for calling Dr Smith's office. This is Carol. How may I help you?" or "Carol speaking."
Welcoming New Patients	
Instead of:	"Do you have an appointment?" or "Yes?"
Use:	"Hello. You must be Mrs. Johnson. My name is Carol. I spoke with you on the telephone. Welcome to our office."
Registering a New Patient	
Instead of:	"Have a seat; fill out these forms. Let me know when you're finished."
Use:	"Mrs. Johnson, it is very important that you fill out both the health and patient registration forms in their entirety. If you have any questions, please let me know. I'm here to help you."
Identifying True Emergencies	
Instead of:	"We're all booked for today."
Use:	"How soon can you be here?" (If the patient has a hair appointment and can't come in until 3:30, this is not a real emergency.)
Scheduling Patients	
Instead of:	"You need another appointment. When do you want to come in?"
Use:	"Mrs. Johnson, Dr. Smith needs to see you again for an hour. Are mornings or afternoons best?" (Always offer the two most difficult times to fill.)

Scheduling Patients	
Instead of:	"See you next time."
Use:	"Mrs. Johnson, we have reserved the doctor's 3:30 p.m. appointment on June 6. We look forward to seeing you then."
Pre-Appointing Hygiene Patients	
Instead of:	"Mrs. Johnson, would you like to go ahead and schedule your six-month check-up?"
Use:	"Mrs. Johnson, if this time of day is good for you, let's go ahead and reserve your preventive care appointment for August."
Confirming Appointments	
Instead of:	"Mrs. Johnson, this is Carol at Dr. Smith's office. I'm calling to remind you of your appointment."
Use:	"Mrs. Johnson, this is Carol at Dr. Smith's office. We're looking forward to seeing you tomorrow at ten."
Rescheduling Patients Who Arrive Late	
Instead of:	"You know you're late. We'll have to reschedule."
Use:	"Mrs. Johnson, thank goodness you're okay. Wait right here to let me see what I can do." Then say, "Our hygienist works on a precise schedule and her next patient is due momentarily. In order to give you the quality of care you deserve, we need to reschedule your appointment."
Many Broken or Changed Appointments in Hygiene	
Instead of:	"Let's go ahead and put your name down in six months. When you get your card, you can change it if the time or date isn't good."
Use:	"Mrs. Johnson, if you choose your appointment time now, you'll have your choice. If you decide not to make an appointment today, when we call you in five months, you'll have to risk not getting a desired appointment time, or our schedule may be completely filled."

Patients Who Choose Not to Schedule Follow-Up Care	
Instead of:	"We'll be glad to file your chart in the inactive files."
Use:	"We are sorry we won't be seeing you on a regular basis. Please keep in mind a telephone call from you is all that is necessary to have you back in our active files. To complete our records, Mrs. Johnson, may I please chart the reason you wish to be inactive?"
Telemarketing Past-Due Patients Whom You've Contacted Several Times	
Instead of:	"Mrs. Johnson, you are overdue for your check-up. Would you like to schedule an appointment?"
Use:	"Mrs. Johnson, we're updating our patient records. Your last appointment with Dr. Smith was (# of months). Your follow-up care is very important. Would you like to make an appointment at this time, or be placed in our inactive files?
"A Meeting Was Called at the Office and I'm Not Going to Be Able to Keep My Appointment in an Hour."	
Instead of:	"Oh, these things happen. We're running behind anyway. When would you like to reschedule?"
Use:	"Oh, I'm sorry, Mrs. Johnson. I know important meetings can be called. Are you sure you can't be here? I had reserved the entire mid-morning just for your appointment. Our assistant Lisa has everything all set up, and the lab is on stand-by to accept your case before lunch today."
Clinical Staff and Collections	
Instead of:	"See you next time."
Use:	"Mrs. Johnson, it was great seeing you today. We'll look forward to your next visit. I've given your chart to Carol. She'll be giving you your receipt for today's visit." Or "I've given your chart to Carol. She'll be processing your insurance immediately and giving you a receipt for the co-payment."

"I Have No Money on Me." "I've Just Written My Last Check." "My Husband Has the Credit Card."	
Instead of:	"That's okay; I'll send a bill."
Use:	(As you hand the patient an envelope with the practice address and postage) "This is our walk-out statement, Mrs. Jones. Please drop your check in the mail tomorrow."
"How Much Is a Crown in Your Office?"	
Instead of:	"We don't quote fees over the phone."
Use:	"Mrs. Johnson, I really cannot answer that question until the doctor has examined your mouth. In order for me to give you a fair estimate, we will need to see you for an examination. Are mornings or afternoons best for you?"
"Why Are Dr. Smith's Fees So Expensive? My Mom's Dentist Only Charges $160 for a Checkup and $625 for a Crown."	
Instead of:	"What's her dentist's name? He must be going broke!" Or, "He doesn't have a very good reputation."
Use:	"Mrs. Johnson, I know you can have your dentistry done less expensively, but after having worked with Dr. Smith the past two years, I also know you can't have it done better."
"My Neighbor's Dentist Only Charges $650 for a Crown. Dr. Smith's Fee is $200 More."	
Instead of:	"I'm sorry, but we just raised our fees."
Use:	"Mrs. Johnson, we would rather apologize for our fees once than the quality of your family's dentistry for a lifetime" or "Only your neighbor's dentist truly knows the value of his/her services. Our fees reflect the quality of ours."

"My Insurance Company Said Your Doctor's Fees Are above Average."	
Instead of:	"I'm not surprised. Everyone's insurance company says that."
Use:	"Mrs. Johnson, as you know, dental insurance companies base their fee schedule on average practices. If we had average fees, we could only provide average care. Dr. Smith wants the best for his patients."
"I'm Sorry I Can't Keep My Appointment. I Have a Terrible Headache and I Just Don't Feel Well."	
Instead of:	"You sound perfectly fine to me. Get dressed and get down here."
Use:	Send a get well card signed by all saying, "Hope you're feeling better." (This will either be excellent public relations or effective at instilling feelings of guilt.)
"I'll Have to Reschedule for Jimmy, Ann, Joe, and Myself Because of Soccer Practice."	
Instead of:	"No problem."
Use:	"Mrs. Johnson, I'm sure you are unaware that we don't normally grant multiple family appointments for this very reason. In the future, we will not be able to schedule all of your family members together."
Patient Only Wants Crown If His Insurance Pays	
Instead of:	"Let's send this off to the insurance company to see what they'll cover."
Use:	"Mr. Johnson, you are one of our lucky patients, as approximately half of your total fee will be paid by your employee benefit plan. I wish all our patients were this fortunate. Many of them must pay the entire fee themselves."

Manage your practice at optimum efficiency and production by generating and then regularly analyzing the data from the reports listed in the table below.

Important Computer Reports	
Report Name	**Data Provided**
Insurance Claim Tracking Report	A list of all insurance filed and what's outstanding by 30, 60, and 90 days.
Production Report	Itemization of service codes, with number rendered, by month and year to date, by provider, and office totals
Payment Report	List of payment sources and dollars (cash, check, credit cards)
Accounts Receivable Report	Summary of accounts receivable and how it is distributed by age…30, 60, 90 days, etc. This can be used for collection tracking. Depending upon vendor, a separate delinquent report with additional collection detail may also be available.
Day Sheet	Listing of charges, payments, and adjustments for the day, by provider, with totals
End of Month Summary	Detail month end totals with year-to-date totals

Report Name	Data Provided
Recare Tracking Report	List of patients due for the month with separate listing for overdue patients in the previous month
Budget Plan-Contract Report	List of patients on each report and their current stages
Referral Tracking Report	Listing of patients who were referred and the referring doctor. This will also provide you with the total dollars expended by patients from a referring source
Treatment Plan Report	Listing of patients with incomplete treatment (treatment presented but not completed)

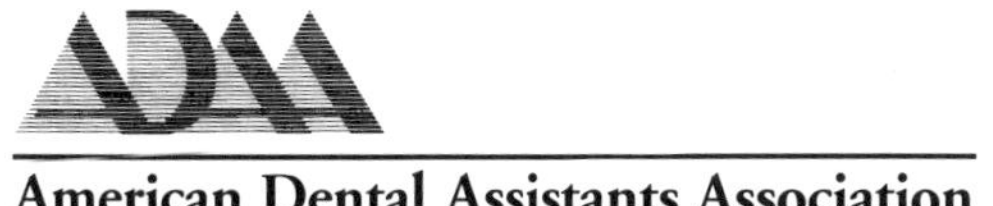

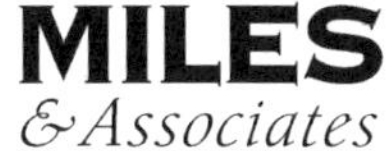

Dear Reader:

We are delighted to have this opportunity to talk to you as you enjoy the many facets of *Dynamic Dentistry*—the textbook—and profit from its content.

Now we have more ways for you to profit from the purchase of this book with the enclosed coupon for trial membership in the American Dental Assistants Association and the Member Appreciation Coupon for those who are already members of ADAA.

Here's how it works.

The trial membership in ADAA will bring you six months of membership in the American Dental Assistants Association with all its benefits.

You'll receive:

- Professional liability insurance
- Additional death and dismemberment insurance
- Discounts on ADAA home study courses and seminars
- Subscription to the *Dental Assistant Journal*
- Free CE in the journal with only a nominal grading fee
- Free subscription to *Dynamic Data Newsletter*—the e-mailed newsletter of Linda L. Miles and Associates
- The knowledge of knowing you are part of America's dedicated dental assisting professionals...the people who make dental assisting a profession!

For those of you who are already ADAA members, we invite you to utilize the coupon for $20.00 worth of continuing education materials as presented in the ADAA professional development catalog. You can visit the catalog online at www.dentalassistant.org or phone for a free copy: 312-541-1550 (fax 312-541-1496). E-mail is ADAA1@aol.com

Librarians and others who have purchased this book—and members of the ADAA—are urged to pass the trial membership along to someone who can profit from it...someone who wants to be part of the people who make dental assisting a profession.

Thank you,

Linda L. Miles, CSP, CMC
CEO

Karen Waide, CDA, EFDA
ADAA President- 2002/2003

35 East Wacker Drive, Suite 1730, Chicago, Illinois 60601-2211
PHONE 312-541-1550 • FAX 312-541-1496 • E-MAIL adaa1@aol.com

DYNAMIC DENTISTRY: PRACTICE MANAGEMENT TOOLS AND STRATEGY FOR BREAKTHROUGH SUCCESS

POST TEST
LM101
5 CEU

1. Dynamic dentistry principles are specifically designed to enable a dental practice to thrive in the ever-changing business and professional environment in which it operates.

a. True
b. False

2. The phrase "Begin with the end in mind" means:

a. Effective people structure their actions around the goals they intend to achieve by the time they are through
b. Effective people structure their choices around the goals they intend to achieve by the time they are through
c. Neither a or b
d. a and b

3. Communication includes:

a. Body language
b. Tone of voice
c. Choice of words
d. Clothes and facial expressions
e. All of the above

4. External communication refers to:

a. Everything that takes place within the practice
b. The messages conveyed to patients and their families and prospective patients
c. None of the above

5. Internal communication refers to:

a. Everything that takes place within the practice
b. The messages conveyed to patients and their families and prospective patients
c. None of the above

6. Regular staff meetings should be held monthly and scheduled during lunch hours.

a. True
b. False

7. Which of the following subjects should never be discussed during treatment time in front of the dental patient?

a. Sex or politics
b. Another employee, doctor, or patient
c. Religion
e. All of the above

8. The word "receptionist" is best replaced by:

a. Business coordinator
b. Scheduling coordinator
c. Patient care facilitator
d. All of the above

9. The tone of one's voice must be:

a. Friendly
b. Knowledgeable
c. Enthusiastic
d. Empathetic
e. a and b
f. All of the above

10. The dynamic dentistry model organizes communication into _____ phases.

a. 2
b. 4
c. 6
d. 8
e. 10

11. Which of the following is/are the "Golden Rule(s)" of dynamic dentistry?

a. Never allow the parent in the treatment room with their children
b. The dental chair cannot go into an upright position until the paper work is completed
c. Never write anything in the chart you wouldn't want the patient to read
d. b and c
e. All of the above

12. Poor or nonexistent teamwork is the root cause of most problems in a dental office.

a. True
b. False

13. The difference between a team and a group of individuals is that a group of individuals:

a. Has members who don't want to share the credit for achievements
b. Is focused on their own needs
c. Focuses on individual goals and individual glory
d. Cannot see a common goal but instead just their own goal
e. b and c
f. All of the above

14. Which of the following is NOT characteristic of a team player:

a. Learns from each other
b. May be threatened by a leader and may therefore undermine the leader's success in big and small ways
c. Sees and believes in a common goal
d. Knows how to make everyone around them perform better
e. Picks each other up

15. DiSC Profile stands for:

a. Dictator, integrity, superior, and constant
b. Dominance, introvert, submissive, and continuity
c. Dominance, image/influence, steadiness, and conscientiousness
d. Dominance, intelligent, steadiness, and conflict

16. How many days is considered to be the recommended trial period to allow the office and the employee adequate time to determine if an applicant is suited for the job?

a. 30 days
b. 60 days
c. 90 days
d. 120 days

17. Nothing is more essential to the smooth, profitable operation of a dental practice than proper patient scheduling.

a. True
b. False

18. The best time to schedule the next appointment is at the end of the present appointment, when the patient is in the office thinking about his or her dental needs and not at home.

a. True
b. False

19. Successful delegating includes:

a. Encouragement to use personal knowledge and skills
b. Expression of confidence
c. Clear and specific instructions
d. Finding the right person for the task
e. All of the above

20. Communication is always aimed at motivating a certain action or set of actions.

a. True
b. False

21. People who call the office as non-emergency new patients should be seen within __________.

a. 24 hours
b. 1 or 2 days
c. 3 or 4 days
d. Middle of the month

22. What is the primary reason dental practices have high accounts receivable?

a. Doctor does not stand behind the office guidelines
b. Lack of collection guidelines
c. Financial coordinator is too busy
d. Staff has never been properly trained

23. A dental practice can have up to a 98% annual collection rate through strong collection policies and practices.

a. True
b. False

24. Which of the following Recare Systems is considered the BEST Recare System in dentistry?

a. No patient ever leaves the office without their next appointment
b. Call and recall system
c. Reminder mailing system

25. Which of the following is/are phases of communication that occur throughout a patient visit?

a. Registration
b. Greeting/welcome
c. Telephone
d. Reappoint and present fee
e. All of the above

ADAA MEMBERSHIP

FREE TRIAL MEMBERSHIP (6 months)

Offer subject to change or cancellation without notice

No copies: only originals will be accepted.

Return this form to:
American Dental Assistants Association
Suite 1730, 35 E. Wacker Drive
Chicago IL 60601-2211

Please print or type and fill all applicable spaces

ADAA member previously? (if yes, when):________ Social Security #________________

Name: ____
LAST FIRST MIDDLE

Street address:______________________________________Apt. #______

City, state, zip: ____

Home phone:____________________ Business phone:____________________

e-mail:________________________________

State Dental Assistants Assn.___ Local Dental Assistants Organization____________

Please specify (if applicable):

CDA #:______________

RDA #:______________

Please check applicable area:

- ☐ Chairside
- ☐ Business Assistant
- ☐ Office Administrator
- ☐ Educator
- ☐ Other ____________________

Signature:______________________________________ Date__________

- Trial Membership may not be used by current ADAA members to renew their membership.
- Membership includes a subscription to *The Dental Assistant,* $50,000 professional dental assisting liability insurance, $2,000 accidental death and dismemberment insurance.
- Membership and professional liability insurance become effective following receipt and processing of application. ADAA insurance becomes effective upon return of a beneficiary card, which will be sent to you with your ADAA membership card.

OFFICE USE ONLY
I______ S______
L______ O______

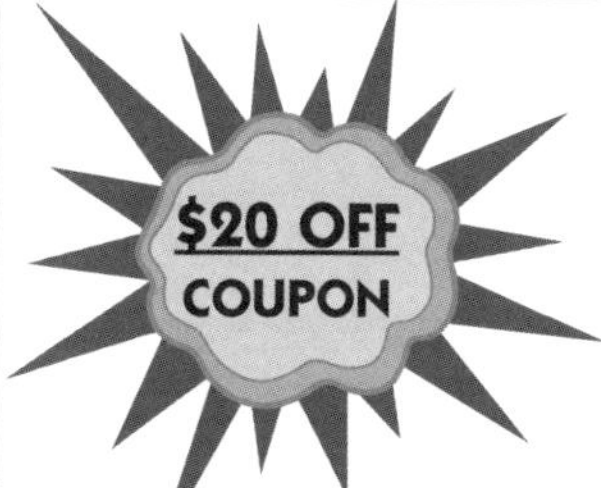

Save on this Promotion *NOW!!!*

ADAA MEMBER APPRECIATION COUPON

Take $20.⁰⁰ off any Continuing Education course

One Coupon Per Course — Offer Expires 12/31/03

Not valid with any other offers or promotions • Shipping based on original amount
This coupon must be presented along with purchase

American Dental Assistants Association, 35 E. Wacker Drive, Suite 1730, Chicago, IL 60601
312/541-1550, ext 211 No copies: only originals will be accepted. *#LM03*

ADAA Test Answer Sheet

FOR OFFICE USE ONLY
Date Received:________
Date Graded:________
Pass Fail:________
Initials:________

"DANB Approval" indicates that a continuing education course appears to meet certain specifications as described in the DANB Recertification Guidelines. DANB does not, however, endorse or recommend any particular continuing education course and is not responsible for the quality of any course content.

DYNAMIC DENTISTRY:

Practice Management Tools and Strategies for Breakthrough Success

Approved for FIVE continuing education credits.

Name:________________________________

Address:________________________________

City, State, Zip:________________________________

Daytime Phone:________________ e-mail:________________

ADAA Membership Number________________

☐ Check or money order for $25 enclosed for non-members.

☐ ADAA member – no grading fee (excluding those with trial membership from this book).

☐ Self-addressed stamped envelope enclosed.

(Completely darken the circle for the correct response)

1. (A) (B) (C) (D) (E) (F)
2. (A) (B) (C) (D) (E) (F)
3. (A) (B) (C) (D) (E) (F)
4. (A) (B) (C) (D) (E) (F)
5. (A) (B) (C) (D) (E) (F)
6. (A) (B) (C) (D) (E) (F)
7. (A) (B) (C) (D) (E) (F)
8. (A) (B) (C) (D) (E) (F)
9. (A) (B) (C) (D) (E) (F)
10. (A) (B) (C) (D) (E) (F)
11. (A) (B) (C) (D) (E) (F)
12. (A) (B) (C) (D) (E) (F)
13. (A) (B) (C) (D) (E) (F)
14. (A) (B) (C) (D) (E) (F)
15. (A) (B) (C) (D) (E) (F)
16. (A) (B) (C) (D) (E) (F)
17. (A) (B) (C) (D) (E) (F)
18. (A) (B) (C) (D) (E) (F)
19. (A) (B) (C) (D) (E) (F)
20. (A) (B) (C) (D) (E) (F)
21. (A) (B) (C) (D) (E) (F)
22. (A) (B) (C) (D) (E) (F)
23. (A) (B) (C) (D) (E) (F)
24. (A) (B) (C) (D) (E) (F)
25. (A) (B) (C) (D) (E) (F)

No copies: only originals will be accepted.

A self-addressed stamped envelope in which you will receive your test results MUST accompany the test when you submit it for grading. Certificate of completion will be included. Tests not accompanied by self-addressed stamped envelope will not be graded or returned. Return this test answer sheet to:

American Dental Assistants Association, Continuing Education Department
35 E. Wacker Drive, Suite 1730, Chicago, IL 60601-2211